.WI

D0969360

THE BIOLOGY OF
A I D S

The Jones and Bartlett Series in Biology

THE BIOLOGY OF
A I D S

SECOND EDITION

HUNG FAN, ROSS F. CONNOR, LUIS P. VILLARREAL
University of California, Irvine

JONES AND BARTLETT PUBLISHERS
BOSTON

Editorial, Sales, and Customer Service Offices
Jones and Bartlett Publishers
20 Park Plaza
Boston, MA 02116

Printed in the United States of America
10 9 8 7 6 5 4 3 2 1

Library of Congress Cataloguing-in-Publication Data

Fan, Hung, 1947-
    The Biology of AIDS / Hung Fan, Ross F. Connor, and Luis P.
    Villarreal. — 2nd ed.
    p.   cm.
    Patterned after a one-quarter course: "AIDS fundamentals" taught
    by the authors at the University of California, Irvine.
    Includes Index
    ISBN 0-86720-178-9
    1. AIDS (Disease) I. Conner, Ross F. II. Villarreal, Luis P. III Title.
[DNLM: 1. Acquired Immunodeficiency Syndrome. WD 308 F199b]
RC607.A26F35 1991
    616.97'92—dc20
DNLM/DLC

    for Library of Congress

                                                    90-15609
                                                        CIP

ACKNOWLEDGMENT

We wish to thank David Fan, Michael Gorman, David Prescott, Cedric Davern, David Baltimore and Frank Lilly for reading the manuscript prior to publication and providing many helpful substantive and editorial comments. Juan Moreno applied outstanding computer graphic skills in generating all the line drawings for the book. Bob Settineri of Sierra Productions was of great help in obtaining the other figures. Maureen Cunningham Neumann and the editorial staff of Jones and Bartlett were responsible for production of the final volume. We wish to thank Michael Feldman, Emmett Carlson and Meridith Peake for their love and support.

DEDICATION

To our HIV-infected friends and acquaintances, who are coura-
geously battling the disease, or who have succumbed to it. In their
honor, and to hasten the day when this book is no longer necessary, a portion of the royalties from this book will be donated to
foundations and community organizations dedicated to AIDS
research and service.

AUTHORS

Dr. Hung Fan is Professor of Virology in the Department of Molecular Biology and Biochemistry at the University of California at Irvine and Director of the UCI Cancer Research Institute. His research interest is in how retroviruses cause disease and induce cancer.

Dr. Ross Conner is Professor of Social Ecology at the University of California, Irvine. Dr. Conner's research interest is in evaluating the effectiveness of public and social programs.

Dr. Luis Villarreal is Professor of Virology in the Department of Molecular Biology and Biochemistry at the University of California, Irvine. Dr. Villarreal's research interest is in the strategy of how viruses replicate and how they cause disease.

PREFACE

The purpose of this text is to provide the nonspecialized student with a firm scientific overview of AIDS from a biomedical perspective. The biological aspects include cellular and molecular descriptions of the immune system and the AIDS virus (Human Immunodeficiency Virus: HIV). The consequences of HIV infection from cell to organism are also covered, along with a clinical description of the disease. As we move from the organism level to the inter-organism level, i.e., the social level, the social ecological aspects of AIDS are also considered. Due to the comprehensive nature of this approach and the additional aim of making this text appropriate for a one-quarter (or semester) course (or part of such a course), these topics can only be covered in a survey fashion. To overcome this limitation, we have selected an approach that focuses first on presenting the relevant fundamental principles. Following a brief presentation of these principles for each particular topic, we then generalize and apply these concepts to the case of AIDS.

This book is patterned after a one-quarter course, "AIDS Fundamentals" at the University of California, Irvine, that is taught by the authors. Approximately one-half of the course covers biomedical aspects of AIDS, and the other part covers social issues raised by the disease. The text represents the material covered in the portion of the course dealing with biomedical aspects; a comprehensive text that includes the social ecology of AIDS is in preparation. At UCI, AIDS Fundamentals is open to all undergraduate students, and is taught assuming that they have had a high school-level modern biology course. The material covered in Chapters 3, 4 and 6 (immunology, virology and epidemiology) is covered in three hours of lecture per chapter. Material covered in the other chapters is taught in a single one-and-a-half hour lecture per chapter. We have found that the students are able to assimilate and retain the material when delivered at this rate.

Most researchers and scholars in AIDS-related fields were unprepared for the dramatic impact of the emerging AIDS epidemic. As virologists and social scientists, we might have expected modern biomedical technology to provide a quick technical solution, or to at least prevent, via vaccine development, the spread of this major new viral epidemic. It is now clear that even though this technology has hastened biomedical progress in AIDS, the AIDS epidemic poses new and unforeseen difficulties with no quick biological solution in sight. These difficulties challenge both our scientific abilities and the ability of our society to respond appropriately. It is our goal to provide the student with a conceptual framework of the issues raised by the AIDS epidemic so that he or she will be better able to deal with the challenges posed by this disease. This is particularly important since new information about scientific aspects of AIDS appears almost daily; with this information comes new implications for the clinical, social, psychological, legal and ethical aspects of the disease. We hope that the framework provided in this book will help the student understand and make informed decisions about AIDS-related issues as they develop in the future.

December, 1990

TABLE OF CONTENTS

THE BIOLOGY OF
A I D S

1

INTRODUCTION: AN OVERVIEW OF AIDS

A Brief Overview of AIDS
The AIDS Epidemic

A REPORT appeared in 1981 that initially drew little attention from infectious disease experts. In that report Dr. Michael Gottlieb, at the University of California at Los Angeles, described a rare form of pneumonia occurring in homosexual men. Other reports about the same time indicated that other homosexual men were developing rare forms of cancer. This new set of symptoms, a syndrome in medical terms, was eventually called *Acquired Immune Deficiency Syndrome* because the symptoms were consistent with damage to the immune system in previously healthy individuals. Moreover, this disease was not congenital or inherited, but appeared to have been acquired. We now know that this resulted from infection by a virus. Since then, the acronym *AIDS*, which is used to describe this disease, has become a prominent and permanent fixture in our language. It evokes a range of human responses, including fear, hate, and mistrust. Some of these responses (hate, mistrust) are related to the association of AIDS with subcultural groups within our society, such as male homosexuals, who already have experienced discrimination. Other responses (fear) are due to the grave nature of the AIDS disease and the threat it may pose to society. This is because the AIDS epidemic continues to grow — unlike most other major infectious diseases that have been controlled by a combination of clinical treatments and public health measures.

A BRIEF OVERVIEW OF AIDS

We now know that AIDS is caused by *Human Immunodeficiency Virus (HIV)*, but it was originally observed by its effects on the immune system. An important clue was that AIDS patients often developed a lung infection (or pneumonia) caused by a fungus called *Pneumocystis carinii*. This infection is very rare in healthy individuals but patients with cancers of the immune system itself (lymphomas) were known to be susceptible to this disease. Lymphomas are usually treated by chemotherapy, which is intended to destroy the cancer cells. However, chemotherapy also will unavoidably destroy many healthy immune cells along with the cancerous lymphoma cells. Thus, this type of pneumonia predominantly occurs in patients with a damaged immune system. Examination of the immune systems in AIDS patients confirmed that their immune systems were damaged. The specific nature of this damage will be discussed in greater detail in Chapters 3 and 4. It had been known for some time that various other virus infections could damage cells of the immune system but such severe damage as seen with AIDS was unprecedented. Although doctors suspected early on that AIDS resulted from infection by a virus, it was not until 1984 that the virus was finally isolated by both French and American researchers. That virus is now known as *HIV*.

In addition to pneumonia, AIDS is associated with numerous other infections. These secondary infections are caused by various bacteria, protozoa, fungi and other viruses. Usually, it is these infections (known as *opportunistic infections*) that cause death in AIDS patients. In addition to secondary infections, AIDS patients frequently develop cancers, including *lymphomas* and an otherwise rare cancer called *Kaposi's sarcoma*. HIV infection also can result in damage to brain cells. This leads to loss of mental function, referred to as AIDS dementia. A more complete description of the clinical features of AIDS is presented in Chapter 5. Most of these opportunistic infections and some other effects of HIV infection can be explained by damage to the immune system by HIV infection.

HIV has a very insidious nature in causing disease. The early stages of infection are often not apparent, without any visible symptoms. The infected person may feel healthy and appear to be completely normal during this time (known as the incubation period) but such a person is able to transmit the infection. The HIV incubation period is of variable duration, and can be quite long (on average 8-10 years). In contrast, for most common virus infections, such as colds or influenza, an incubation period of a few days or weeks will be closely followed by apparent disease. This adds greatly to the difficulty in studying and controlling AIDS, because many people who are infected with the virus have not yet developed the disease.

THE AIDS EPIDEMIC

Despite the many different clinical symptoms that result from AIDS, medical investigators have already learned a great deal about how AIDS is spread in our population. For example, it is now clear that HIV transmission requires close contact and that infection occurs by one of only three routes: blood, birth, or sex. Casual contact does not lead to disease transmission. AIDS epidemiology will be further discussed in Chapter 6.

Between 1981 (the beginning of AIDS epidemic) and the end of 1989 about 120,000 cases of AIDS have been reported to the National Center for Disease Control (CDC) in Atlanta, Georgia. Of these cases, about 71,000 (60%) have died. Sexually active homosexual males were originally the major afflicted group and represent about 60% of these reported cases. Another 21% of the cases were male or female intravenous drug users, and 7% were both male homosexuals and drug users. The remaining 12% resulted either from heterosexual transmission, birth, or by blood transfusion during the period when American blood supply was not monitored for HIV antibodies (1981-1985).

The AIDS epidemic is not restricted to the United States of America. It can be found in all continents and hence is considered a pandemic. There may be as many as ten million people in subsaharan Africa who are infected with HIV. In Africa, HIV transmission predominantly results from heterosexual contact, and other modes as well. Given the relatively poor medical support available in much of Africa, the number of infected people may increase significantly. As there is no current cure for AIDS these numbers are alarming. They indicate the clear potential of AIDS to spread unchecked, in spite of recent advances in modern medicine, epidemiology, virology, and recombinant DNA technology. This reminds us of previous times when major infectious diseases devastated human populations (see Chapter 2). How can we control this epidemic? An overview of the relationship between epidemics and human populations may shed some light on this, as discussed in the next chapter.

2

CONCEPTS OF INFECTIOUS DISEASE AND A HISTORY OF EPIDEMICS

Factors that affect Spread of Epidemics
- Host and Virus Populations
- The Transmission Rate
- Population Densities and Infections
- Controlling Infectious Diseases

A History of Epidemics
- The Old World
- The New World
- Modern Concepts of Infectious Disease
- Epidemics in Modern Times
- Syphilis: The Social Problems with a Sexually Transmitted Disease

O NE OF THE GREAT recent achievements of modern civilization has been the control of infectious diseases. It is likely that few of us personally know someone who died from a contagious disease. In historical terms, however, this is a new development, which occurred in this century. In previous centuries death due to infectious diseases was common, and whole populations were often affected.

When a population becomes infected with a contagious disease an *epidemic* results. "Epidemic" is derived from Greek, and means "in one place among the people." To understand how an infectious disease can spread or remain established in a population we must consider the relationship between an infectious disease agent and its host population. The study of diseases in populations is an area of medicine known as epidemiology, which will be further discussed in Chapter 6.

We now know that contagious diseases are spread by microorganisms such as certain bacteria and viruses, that cause disease when they infect a susceptible person. This is a modern concept, known as the *germ theory* of infectious disease. As we shall see, earlier societies often used moral or religious explanations for infectious disease, and their societal behavior reflected those beliefs.

FACTORS THAT AFFECT SPREAD OF EPIDEMICS

HOST AND VIRUS POPULATION. An epidemic consists of infection of a number of individuals in a population. It is important to look at more than a single person in understanding how diseases spread. Two populations must be considered. One population is that of human host and the other is the infecting agent — in the case of AIDS, a virus. These two populations have a parasite-host relationship, or a predator-prey relationship, where the human population is the prey and the virus is the predator. Just as a predator can deplete its prey, a viral infection can also deplete or limit the population of its host. For example, a lethal virus that spreads rapidly might kill all available hosts, leading to the extinction of both its host and itself. The outcome of an epidemic, however, is not always straightforward and can vary according to a number of other factors that relate to the population. These factors include:

1) the total number of hosts;
2) their birth rate;
3) the number of susceptible hosts who are not infected;
4) the rate at which the disease can be transmitted from an infected individual to an uninfected one;
5) the number of infected individuals who die;
6) the number who survive the infection and become immune or resistant to further infection.

Figure 2-1 shows a schematic relationship between infected and uninfected people and summarizes the above factors. The arrows that connect the boxed groups represent movement of people from one group to an adjacent one. This scheme is a simplified representation of the dynamics or "ecology" of a virus epidemic. It is possible to develop mathematical models to describe or predict an epidemic if the rates of movement through the scheme can be determined. One of the applications of the field of epidemiology (see Chapter 6) is to determine these rates.

THE TRANSMISSION RATE. The arrow in Figure 2-1 that connects the susceptibles to the infected group is the *transmission rate*

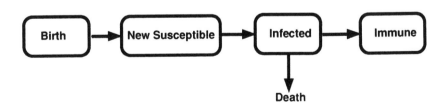

FIGURE 2-1. Population factors that affect epidemics:
1. Population size;   2. Birth rate;   3. Number of susceptibles;
4. Transmission rate;   5. Death rate;   6. Immune rate.

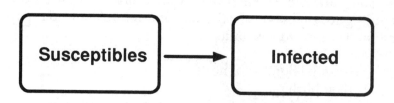

FIGURE 2-2. Transmission rate of infections:
1. Inherent efficiency of virus infection;
2. Encounter rate between infected and uninfected.

of infection. This *rate* represents the efficiency at which disease is transmitted from an infected to a susceptible person. This transmission rate has two major components (Figure 2-2). One of these components is the inherent efficiency with which a specific virus can infect a susceptible person. The inherent efficiency will depend on the specific virus being considered as well as other factors, such as the route by which the virus enters the susceptible person. For example, measles virus, like many other respiratory viruses, has a high inherent efficiency of transmission and is therefore highly contagious. HIV on the other hand, actually has a relatively poor inherent transmission efficiency.

The other major component of the transmission rate is the rate at which a susceptible person encounters an infectious person. Each encounter between an infected and uninfected person increases the likelihood that an infection will be transmitted.

As we shall see later with the AIDS virus, both of these components of transmission can be changed by altering the behavior of susceptible and infected persons. Behaviors that allow high encounter rates with infected people or that allow more efficient infection will favor the spread of an epidemic. Conversely, changes in behavior that reduce these transmission factors may control the spread of an epidemic.

POPULATION DENSITIES AND INFECTIONS. Many of the epidemics that have plagued mankind for the last few thousand years would not have had a favorable transmission rate during early human civilization. Early human societies were not urban, but consisted of hunter-gatherers who lived in relatively small groups such as extended families. Such small groups or small populations cannot produce new susceptibles in high enough numbers at any given time to support the continued occurrence of many epidemic diseases. An acute disease will produce symptoms and make a person infectious soon after infection. The infected person will either transmit the disease, die from the infection, or recover and become immune to subsequent infections. An acute epidemic that strikes such small groups will quickly infect all available susceptibles, then die out.

About 10,000 years ago the agricultural revolution allowed human populations to become large enough to support epidemics. In other words, the development of human civilization was necessary before epidemics by acute disease could establish stable footholds. When the world population became sufficiently large, different patterns of infection could also develop. Epidemic diseases could establish an *endemic* pattern — one in which the disease is always present. Following the initial introduction and spread into a suggestible or naive population, even a very lethal disease can become endemic. In an endemic disease, the numbers who are actively infected are much lower, but the disease is always present in the population. Generally, endemic diseases are childhood diseases because the virus is so common in the population that individuals encounter it during childhood. Most adults have had the disease and survived. This may account for much of the high infant mortality of previous eras (Europe in the Dark and Middle Ages), and of high infant mortality in some developing countries today. By selecting for survivors, endemic infectious agents can limit population sizes and result in populations that are relatively unaffected or resistant to the infectious agent as a whole. As we shall see in the following pages, this can have major historical consequences when two previously separated societies encounter each other for the first time. It is also likely that endemic and epidemic diseases have had a major effect on social development, since there is an important behavioral component in the efficiency of infection spread.

In addition to acute diseases such as measles, there are also chronic infections. In acute infections, the disease symptoms generally occur quite soon after infection, and the infectious agent is generally eliminated after the initial disease period. In a chronic infection, the person does not eliminate the infectious agent (often a virus). The virus persists in the infected person and may be produced at low levels. Chronic infections will often not show symptoms or disease immediately after infection. As described above, acute infections generally require large populations (with continued new susceptibles) in order to be maintained. In contrast, chronic infections can sometimes be maintained in small populations. In addition, chronic infections are often more difficult to control because infected and uninfected people may be indistinguishable. As we shall see below, the syphilis epidemic was difficult to control partly because syphilis is a chronic infection. Like syphilis, AIDS is also a chronic infection.

CONTROLLING INFECTIOUS DISEASES. Since the turn of this century there has been a steady and dramatic decrease in the number of people who die from infectious diseases. Recently most modern developed countries have been free of major lethal contagious diseases. For bacterial diseases, antibiotics can kill the infections after they start. Viruses pose a different problem: they are difficult to eliminate once they become established. Therefore, viral diseases have been controlled mostly by vaccination (see Chapter 4), but occasionally by other measures. A vaccine interrupts the flow of new susceptibles from newborns into the susceptible sub-population by making young people immune without ever spreading infectious virus (Figure 2-3). If enough (but not necessarily all) susceptibles become immunized, this confers immunity to the population as a whole. This is because the remaining un-immunized but susceptible individuals are unlikely to encounter another infectious individual. It is possible to eliminate some diseases completely from the human population with an effective vaccination program. The smallpox virus, that was responsible for so much human death in historic times, is now extinct due to successful worldwide vaccination efforts.

A HISTORY OF EPIDEMICS

THE OLD WORLD. Even the very earliest historical records document the major impact of epidemics. It is not always clear to us now which infectious agent was causing a particular epidemic in ancient times, but we can often make guesses from the recorded symptoms. The three disease agents that have probably caused most human deaths are smallpox virus, measles virus, and the plague bacterium, *Yersinia pestis*. These three diseases have accounted for hundreds of millions of human deaths over the years and an unfathomable amount of human suffering. Other important epidemic agents include influenza virus, typhoid fever bacterium, yellow fever virus, polio virus, and more recently hepatitis virus. The syphilis bacterium *Treponema pallidum* is of special interest, due to its sexual mode of transmission and its associated social problems. Many historical accounts make clear reference, however, to a supposed religious or moral reason for a particular epidemic. The transmission of disease itself was often believed to occur through casting of an "evil eye." In the Old Testament, for example, Moses brought onto the Egyptians a plague of "sores that break into pustules" due to the "willfulness" of the Pharaoh. Epidemics were often perceived as punishment due to the wrath of a deity, perhaps for some offence by the entire population.

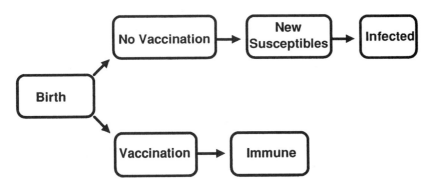

FIGURE 2-3. Epidemic control by vaccination.

Those who developed a disease were viewed as deserving it. This tendency to link a disease to social stigmatism has persisted throughout history, and afflicts people with AIDS today.

The Greek writings are probably the earliest accounts in sufficient detail to allow us to measure the impact of epidemic disease. Aside from malaria, the Greeks were relatively free of most infectious diseases with one important exception. In 430-429 B.C. an epidemic that may have been measles struck Athens with a devastating loss of life. It also resulted in a significant decrease in the size of its armies — and the following year Athens lost a war with Sparta. Thus, this epidemic may have influenced history.

The Roman Empire also suffered massive epidemics in 165 A.D. and again in 251 A.D. Prior to the 165 A.D. epidemic, population of the Roman Empire was probably at its peak (about 54 million). After the 164 A.D. and 251 A.D. epidemics, Roman population did not recover its size until modern times. The first epidemic was possibly smallpox, and appears to have killed one third of Rome's population. The 251 A.D. epidemic may have been due to measles, and was equally devastating; there were about 5,000 deaths per day in Rome at its peak. Rome's rural population may have been even more affected. This die-off may have led to depopulation of agricultural lands and an inability to oppose invasion from the north. A third massive epidemic occurred in 542-543 A.D., probably due to Bubonic Plague. Soon after this plague, Rome's armies fell to the Visigoth and then the Moslem armies, and the Dark Ages of Europe began. Thus, epidemiological history suggests that infectious diseases may have contributed to the fall of the Roman Empire. The situation for the Han Chinese society, although more difficult to estimate, appears to have been similar. Massive epidemics in 162 A.D. and again in 310 A.D. may account for much of the population decline in China, which peaked at about 50 million at those times, but declined to about 8.9 million by 742 A.D.

In Europe, and probably also in China, measles and smallpox eventually became endemic childhood diseases following these devastating epidemics. In the following millennia, Europe experienced still further devastating epidemics known as the Black Death. Black Death was a pneumonic form (or lung infection) of plague, which had a very high fatality rate. It probably accounted for up to 100 million deaths in Europe. The worst of these epidemics occurred in 1346. This epidemic appears to have been a *pandemic*, meaning that other continents (China and India) were also involved. The Black Death recurred in Europe in the 1360s and again in the 1370s. The seemingly arbitrary pattern of death, and the massive suffering had dark social consequences for Europe. Xenophobia, the fear of foreigners, became common. Violent riots against Jews and Gypsies occurred in numerous cities as they were blamed as a source of the plague. Self-flagellation became a common practice and rational theology lost popular acceptance. The situation improved somewhat in the 1400s. Black Death became endemic, possibly because of selection for a less virulent plague bacterium; selection for people with greater resistance to the disease also may have occurred. European society was now experiencing most of these various acute infectious diseases, especially the viral diseases, as childhood diseases.

THE NEW WORLD. A well-documented example of what happens when a new viral disease enters a naive population occurred when Cortez came to Mexico and introduced smallpox into the New World. The Aztec Codices (hieroglyphic-like records) tell us that the new world was relatively free of major infectious disease at that time. The population of Mexico was probably 25-30 million, and Mexico City may have then been the most populous city in the world. In 1518, just as the Aztecs drove Cortez from Mexico City, a smallpox epidemic swept though the city, killing the Aztec leaders and decimating the city's population. This epidemic was followed by numerous other diseases that were endemic European childhood diseases, but devastating to the Aztecs. Within 50 years, the population of Mexico was down to about 1.5 million, or about 5% of what it had been at its peak. Furthermore, the fact that the diseases seemed only to strike the Aztecs and not the Spaniards, led the Aztecs to believe that the Gods favored the Spaniards.

Other American natives fared even worse than the Aztecs: the Indians of Baja California and other island tribes became totally extinct. Thus, the main fabric of native American society was utterly destroyed. Mexico's population only began to recover in the 1800s, and only now has Mexico City become the most populous city in the world again. A similar fate was in store for the Pacific island natives, who also suffered huge population losses after encountering European explorers. Thus, throughout human history infectious diseases have profoundly affected human populations.

MODERN CONCEPTS OF INFECTIOUS DISEASE. The germ theory of infection was first proposed in 1546 by Girolamo Fracatoro, a Franciscan monk. However, it was not until the 1840s that H. Henle, a German physician, clarified these concepts and they became accepted among scientists. One of Henle's students, Robert Koch, subsequently proposed four postulates that could be used to prove that an infectious agent causes a disease. This was a historic milestone in the concepts of infectious disease. Koch's postulates state that an organism can be considered to cause a disease if it fulfills the following criteria:

1. The organism is always found in diseased individuals.
2. The organism can be isolated from the diseased individual and grown pure in culture.
3. The pure culture will initiate and reproduce the disease when introduced back into a susceptible host (either man or animal).
4. The organism must be re-isolated from the diseased individual.

These postulates allowed scientifically sound assignments of which agents caused specific diseases, and freed physicians from many superstitions and myths that had historically prevailed.

Actually by today's standards Koch's postulates are sometimes too stringent. For example, viruses cannot be grown pure in culture in the absence of cells (see Chapter 4). Also, if two infectious agents cooperate to cause a disease or a particular set of symptoms, it would also be impossible to fulfill Koch's postulates. (We shall see that this situation applies to HIV infection and AIDS.) In the late 1800s, however, such stringency was necessary.

The timing of the development of Koch's postulates and of the development of the science of epidemiology was most fortunate, because other changes in society set the stage for the outbreak of another worldwide epidemic. In the late 1800s steamships brought about relatively rapid world travel. This change impacted the ecology of infectious disease by allowing the rapid movement of infected persons who could quickly spread an epidemic. In 1894 another plague pandemic broke out, initially in Burma, then in Hong Kong, then via steamships to all major ports worldwide, including those in the United States. By applying the germ theory of disease and epidemiology, society was able to respond to this threat. The application of Koch's postulates led to the rapid identification and isolation of the causative bacteria, *Yersinia pestis*. Furthermore, intense epidemiological studies identified rats, and more specifically their fleas, as major carriers of the disease. This led to development of preventative measures to control the spread of the plague, principally by limiting interactions between rats and humans. Except for a further breakout in India, the plague epidemic was stopped. This was an important lesson. There was no cure or vaccine for plague at this time, yet changes in human behavior designed to minimize infection averted a pandemic. With the current AIDS epidemic we are in a similar situation, because there is currently no cure or vaccine. However, because AIDS is predominantly a sexually transmitted disease, modification of behavior to control its spread will be more difficult.

EPIDEMICS IN MODERN TIMES. In the twentieth century several other epidemics have taken a toll on humanity. During the great pandemic of 1918, Influenza virus killed about 20 million people worldwide and virtually brought World War I to a halt. About 80% of American casualties in World War I were due to Influenza, a fact seldom mentioned in most history texts. Influenza continues to cause epidemics and remains a health threat. The major reason is because this virus can mutate rapidly. These mutations lead to changes in the surface structure of the virus, which allow the virus to avoid the protection of the immune system. As a result, individuals who were previously infected with Influenza virus are not protected from the new mutant virus. As we will see later, HIV also has a similar property.

Polio virus is another recent epidemic disease. This disease appeared as a "new" viral epidemic in the United States in 1894 — much like the way the AIDS epidemic appeared in 1981. Polio virus can damage the nervous system and lead to paralysis. Although polio virus had been infecting people since early history it probably did not cause epidemics until 1894. We now believe that improvements in hygiene and sanitation occurring in more developed societies actually predisposed individuals to the paralytic form of polio by delaying exposure to the virus until they were young adults. Infection of infants, which tends to occur in developing countries, usually results in a mild non-paralytic gastrointestinal infection. Thus, the people most likely to get paralytic polio were the healthy young adults from the highest socio-economic classes. This demonstrates the unforeseen effect that changes in social behavior can have on the ecology of an epidemic. This disease had a major impact on the American consciousness, as seen by highly visible national crusades during the first half of the twentieth century (the March of Dimes). This underlines the way that the nature of the victims can profoundly influence public perceptions of a disease, and also society's response to it. In fact, there were about 50,000 total deaths from paralytic polio during the first half of this century. It is interesting to contrast the public response to polio during this time to recent responses to AIDS — even though as many deaths from AIDS have occurred in less than ten years.

SYPHILIS: THE SOCIAL PROBLEMS WITH A SEXUALLY TRANSMITTED DISEASE. One epidemic that is hauntingly similar to the AIDS epidemic is syphilis. The parallels are striking. At the time of the syphilis epidemic, scientific investigation of this insidious disease was at the leading edge of medicine and microbiology, similar to the current situation with AIDS. The issues raised included public health policy and civil liberties, again as in the AIDS epidemic. And finally, because it was a sexually transmitted disease, syphilis patients were highly stigmatized. A cure for syphilis in infected individuals was developed in 1909, but it was not until the 1940s that the epidemic was finally controlled.

Why did it take so long to control this epidemic? Like AIDS, syphilis can be a long-term and variable disease, with phases in which no symptoms are apparent. Unfortunately, untreated syphilis often eventually leads to death. More important, at the time, syphilis was perceived as a social problem — hence the reference to it as a "social" disease. Many blamed the disease on a breakdown of social values, and promoted the view that a sexual ethic in which all sex was marital and monogamous would make it impossible to acquire the disease. The initial public health policies to control this epidemic were based on these views. Abstinence from extramarital sexual contact was encouraged and prostitution was repressed, since prostitutes were blamed as the major source of infection of otherwise monogamous males. Immigrants were also blamed for bringing the disease from abroad, even though epidemiological data did not support this view. As many as 20,000 prostitutes were quarantined or jailed during World War I. In addition, the Army discouraged the availability of condoms for fear that they might encourage extramarital sex by soldiers. There were also campaigns to dishonor soldiers who became infected with syphilis by giving them a dishonorable discharge. These policies were not based on epidemiologic evidence, and they failed to control the epidemic, which actually grew during this period.

It was not until the 1930s that the surgeon general of the United States, Thomas Parren, proposed major changes in the public health approaches to control the syphilis epidemic. These policy changes were ultimately successful but required substantial funding from Congress. These proposals called for the elimination of repressive approaches that discouraged people from participating in programs or seeking treatment. Free and confidential diagnostic and treatment centers were set up throughout the nation. A national educational campaign was begun to educate the public and dispel prevalent misconceptions (even among respected sources) about its transmission. Syphilis is transmitted by sexual contact, but not casual contact. These policies, along with new antibiotics brought the syphilis epidemic under control in the 1940s.

With the AIDS epidemic we are dealing with powerful biological drives, such as human sexuality, and drug addiction. The syphilis epidemic shows us that repressive policies based mainly on abstinence are not very effective in controlling a sexually transmitted disease. Other alterations in behavior will be necessary to reduce the transmission of AIDS and bring this epidemic under control. Until a cure or a vaccine against AIDS is developed, changing behavior is our most effective means of controlling the AIDS pandemic.

3

THE IMMUNE SYSTEM

A S MENTIONED in Chapter 1, AIDS results from a viral infection that ultimately disables the immune system. In order to understand this disease we need to understand the immune system. This system is an intricate collection of cells and fluids in our body that gives us the ability to fight off infections. HIV, the AIDS virus, specifically affects certain cells of the immune system. Once we know about these cells and what they do, we can then see how HIV does its damage. This chapter provides a simplified overview of immunity — many more intricacies and details are known, but the information provided here will allow us to understand the basic immunological problems associated with AIDS.

Blood

In order to understand the immune system, we must first consider blood. Blood is a system of circulating cells and fluids that carries out many important functions for the body. These functions include: 1) *transport of nutrients and oxygen* to the body tissues; 2) *elimination of waste products and carbon dioxide* from tissues; 3) *wound repair;* and 4) *protection from infection by foreign agents.* Besides cells, the fluid portion of blood contains many different substances and molecules that help carry out these functions. Some examples are sugars that are necessary for energy metabolism in our tissues, and antibodies, which are important in fighting infections. The cell-free fluid portion of blood is referred to as plasma or serum. Serum can be obtained from isolated blood by letting it stand and clot; the cells are trapped in the clot and can be removed easily.

Cells and substances of the blood that are responsible for protection from infection make up the *immune system*. The immune system must protect us from a wide variety of infectious agents. These include (in ascending order of complexity):

Viruses. These are very small subcellular agents — (see Chapter 4).

Bacteria. These are small single cell microorganisms that have relatively simple genetic material.

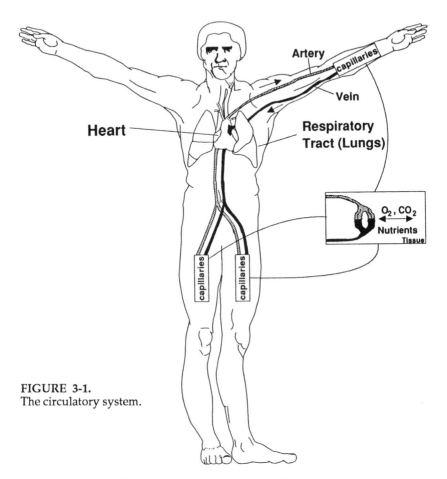

FIGURE 3-1.
The circulatory system.

Protozoa. These are large single-cell microorganisms that contain more complicated genetic structures. Amoebas and Giardia are examples of protozoa.

Fungi. These are more complex microorganisms that may exist as single cells, or they may be organized into simple multicellular organisms. Examples are yeasts and molds.

Multicellular Parasites. These can be relatively large organisms, such as roundworms and tape worms.

In addition, the immune system is also important in fighting cancer.

Blood is carried throughout the body by a series of blood vessels that make up the *circulatory system* (Figure 3-1). The heart is the pump for the circulatory system, and it moves blood through the blood vessels by its rhythmic muscular contractions. There are three kinds of blood vessels: 1) *arteries,* which carry blood away from the heart to the body tissues; 2) *veins,* which carry blood back to the heart from the tissues; and 3) *capillaries.* Capillaries are very thin-walled blood vessels in the tissues that connect the arteries with the veins, and they allow exchange of oxygen, nutrients, and wastes between the blood and tissues. Some kinds of blood cells (such as white blood cells called monocytes and lymphocytes — refer page 26) can also pass through these thin walls from the blood into the tissues as well. The lungs are another important part of the circulatory system — this is where exchange of oxygen and carbon dioxide between the blood and the air we breathe takes place.

The cells in the blood have limited life spans — ranging from one or two days to several weeks depending on the cell type. This means that they must be replenished continually. They are replenished from *stem cells* that are located in the bone marrow. These stem cells have the capacity 1) to divide and make more of themselves, and 2) to differentiate and mature into blood cells of all types (Figure 3-2). During the differentiation process the stem cells first develop into committed precursors, which can either divide or differentiate into mature blood cells of a particular kind. This process goes on throughout life, and, if interrupted, results in very serious health problems.

When stem cells and committed precursors divide or differentiate, they require the presence of *growth factors* in order to carry out these processes. Different growth factors stimulate particular kinds of blood cells; these growth factors play important roles in regulating the orderly growth and replenishment of all blood cells. For example, interleukin 2 is a growth factor that is required by blood cells called T-lymphocytes — more about this later.

CELLS OF THE BLOOD. Let us now look at the different kinds of cells present in blood. These cells are shown in Figure 3-3. Blood cells are divided into *red blood cells* and *white blood cells.* There are a lot of red blood cells, but they are a single cell type; the white

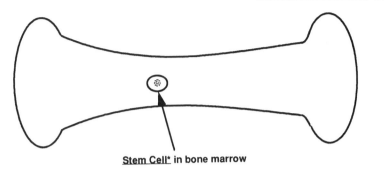

Stem Cell* in bone marrow

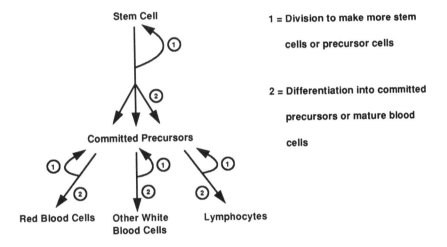

Stem Cell

1 = Division to make more stem cells or precursor cells

2 = Differentiation into committed precursors or mature blood cells

Committed Precursors

Red Blood Cells

Other White Blood Cells

Lymphocytes

FIGURE 3-2. Growth and maturation of blood cells.

blood cells are fewer in number, but they are made up of many cell types.

Red blood cells or erythrocytes are responsible for carrying oxygen to the tissues and carbon dioxide away from them. They contain a protein called hemoglobin that binds and carries the oxygen or carbon dioxide within them. Hemoglobin gives red blood cells their characteristic red color. All of the other blood cells are called white blood cells, since they lack hemoglobin.

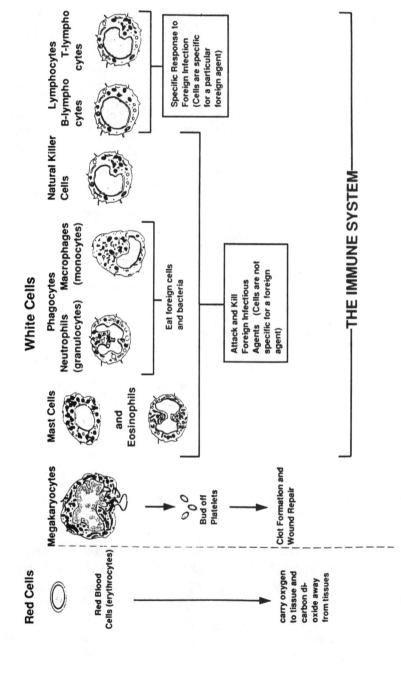

FIGURE 3-3. Cells of the blood.

White blood cells or leukocytes:

Megakaryocytes are very large blood cells that bud off subcellular particles called *platelets*. Platelets circulate through the blood stream, and if they encounter a break in a blood vessel they cause a clot to form. Thus they are involved in *wound repair*.

Cells of the immune system. There are two classes of cells in the immune system: those that respond to a specific foreign agent or substance, and those that are *not* specific for the agent they attack. The cells that are specific for a certain foreign agent are *lymphocytes*. Cells that are not specific for the foreign agent they attack include *phagocytes*, *mast cells, eosinophils* and *natural killer cells*.

Phagocytes are cells that attack and eliminate foreign cells or bacteria by engulfing or "eating" them. In fact, *phagein* is the Greek word meaning "to eat." There are two different kinds of phagocytes: *macrophages* (also called monocytes) and *neutrophils* (also called phagocytic granulocytes). Macrophages generally attack and engulf cells infected with viruses, while neutrophils generally attack foreign bacteria.

Mast cells and *eosinophils* attack infectious agents that are too large to be engulfed by a single blood cell. Such agents include protozoa and large parasites such as worms. Mast cells and eosinophils come into contact with the foreign agents and release toxic compounds that may kill those foreign agents.

What instructs phagocytes, mast cells and eosinophils to attack a foreign agent? In general, *antibodies*, which are proteins produced by certain lymphocytes, first bind to the foreign agent in a specific fashion. The phagocytes, mast cells or eosinophils then recognize the agent because of the antibodies bound to it, and they attack. This process is diagramed in Figure 3-4.

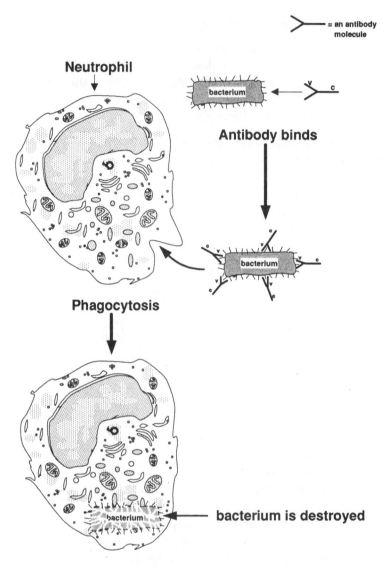

FIGURE 3-4. The action of phagocytes.

Lymphocytes are cells that respond *specifically* to particular foreign substances. In this regard, it is important to define an *antigen*. An antigen is a molecule or substance against which lymphocytes will raise a response. An example of an antigen would be a protein of a virus particle; the number of possible antigens that we might encounter is virtually limitless.

Lymphocytes are divided into two types: *B-lymphocytes* and *T-lymphocytes*. *B-lymphocytes* secrete soluble proteins called *antibodies* into the circulatory system. Each individual antibody specifically recognizes and binds to one particular antigen. Once this happens the antibody signals other cells in the immune system to attack (Figure 3-4). In addition, certain antibodies may bind directly and inhibit the function of infectious agents such as viruses.

T-lymphocytes (or T-cells) make proteins called *receptors* that are similar to antibodies, in that these proteins recognize specific antigens. However, T-lymphocytes do not release their receptors, but hold them on their cell surfaces. As a result, the T-lymphocytes themselves specifically recognize and bind to foreign antigens.

There are two major kinds of T-lymphocytes: *Cytotoxic* or *killer* T-cells (T_{killer}), and *Helper* T-cells (T_{helper}). T_{killer} cells directly bind cells carrying a foreign antigen. Once they bind to them, they attack and kill those cells, thus eliminating them from the body. T_{helper} cells, on the other hand, do not kill cells. Instead, they interact with B-lymphocytes or T_{killer} lymphocytes and "help" them respond to antigens — more about this later. In addition to the receptors, T_{killer} and T_{helper} cells each have characteristic proteins on their surfaces: the *CD8* protein is present on T_{killer} cells, and the *CD4* protein is present on T_{helper} cells (Figure 3-5). Simple tests have been devised for the CD4 and CD8 proteins, and they can be used for identifying and counting T_{killer} and T_{helper} lymphocytes.

T-lymphocytes get their name from the fact that their maturation depends on passage through the thy-

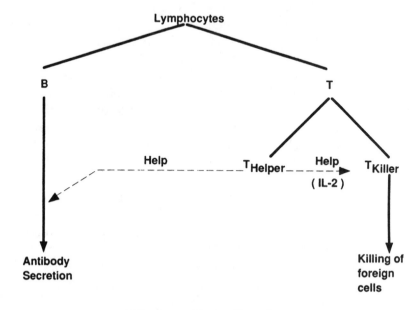

FIGURE 3-5. Kinds of lymphocytes.

mus gland. The thymus is a butterfly-shaped gland that lies over the heart.

Natural killer cells are cells that resemble T-lymphocytes in many physical properties, although they also show some differences. These cells attack virus-infected cells and tumor cells and kill them. Natural killer cells exist in normal individuals who have not previously encountered the infectious agent or cancer — this is different from the situation for B- and T-lymphocytes as we shall see. Furthermore, individual natural killer cells are not specific for the cells that they attack, which also distinguishes them from B- and T-lymphocytes.

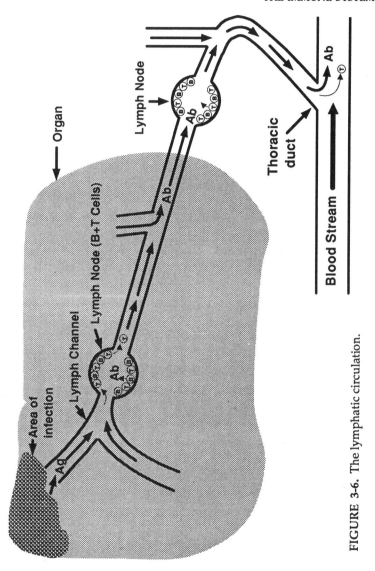

FIGURE 3-6. The lymphatic circulation.

The Lymphatic Circulation

Lymphocytes (both B-cells and T-cells) circulate through the blood vessels, and also through a second circulatory system, the *lymphatic circulation*. The lymphatic circulation is made up of *lymph channels* in our tissues, which drain lymph fluid from the tissues into structures called *lymph nodes* (Figure 3-6). The lymph nodes contain B-lymphocytes and T-lymphocytes, which can respond to foreign antigens during infections. As an example, suppose a tissue becomes infected with a microorganism such as a virus. Pieces of virus or whole virus particles will be transported in the lymph fluid down the lymph channels to the lymph node. In the lymph node the virus may be recognized as an antigen by B- or T-lymphocytes. These cells respond by secretion of antibodies specific for the virus (B-cells), or production of T-lymphocytes specific for the virus. These antibodies and lymphocytes are then drained from the lymph node through another lymph channel, which joins other lymph channels from other parts of the tissue. Ultimately, fluid from lymph channels from all over the body is collected together and emptied into a main vessel called the thoracic duct, which empties into the blood stream. As a result, antibodies and lymphocytes that are produced in response to an infection at one site or tissue will be distributed by the blood stream throughout the body.

During infections the lymph nodes near the site of the infection frequently become enlarged. This is because the lymphocytes in these lymph nodes are dividing rapidly and producing large amounts of antibody and cells to fight the infectious agent. You may have noticed "swollen glands" in your neck if you get some respiratory infections. This is an example of this process.

B-CELLS AND HUMORAL IMMUNITY: THE GENERATION OF ANTIBODIES. Let us now look at how B-lymphocytes respond to a foreign antigen by making antibodies. This part of the immune system is referred to as *humoral immunity*, since it results in production of antibodies that circulate in the blood stream. "Humor" is derived from the Latin word for "fluid."

An antibody molecule is made up of four proteins that are bound together: two of these proteins are identical and are called *heavy chains*; the other two are also identical and are called *light chains*. A protein is a linear chain of building block molecules called *amino acids* — much like beads on a string. There are twenty possible amino acids, and the nature of a protein is determined by the particular sequence of these twenty amino acids that it contains (Figure 3-7). In the case of antibodies, the two heavy chain

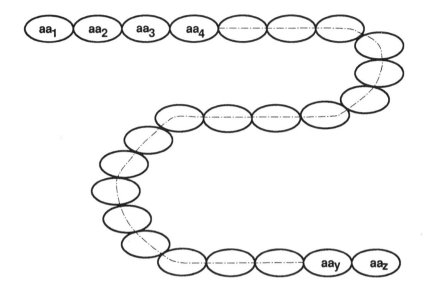

aa$_1$= amino acid number 1 in the protein chain

aa$_2$= amino acid number 2 in the protein chain

etc.

FIGURE 3-7. Protein structure.

proteins are larger than the two light chain proteins. These proteins are held together by chemical bonding into a Y-shaped molecule, as shown in Figure 3-8. Each antibody molecule is specific for one particular antigen, and this specificity is determined by the sequence of amino acids in the light and heavy chains. If several different antibodies with different specificities are compared, certain regions of the light and heavy chains are very similar for the different antibodies. These regions are referred to as *constant regions* or C-regions. Other parts of the light and heavy chain proteins are different for each different antibody in terms of the amino acid building block sequence. These parts are called the *variable regions* or V-regions. In terms of the function

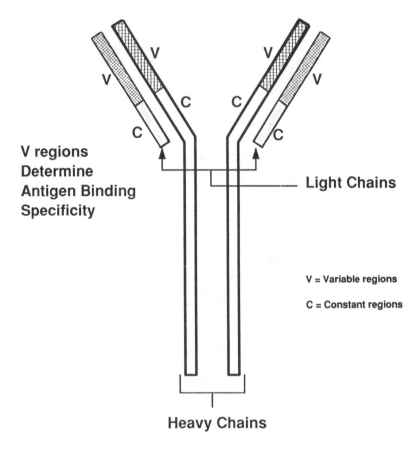

V regions Determine Antigen Binding Specificity

Light Chains

V = Variable regions

C = Constant regions

Heavy Chains

FIGURE 3-8. Structure of an antibody molecule.

of the antibody, the protein sequences of the variable regions determine which antigen the antibody will bind to. An antibody will "fit" its antigen similar to how a key fits only its own lock. Once an antibody is bound to its proper antigen, the C-regions then signal other parts of the immune system to attack — for instance, phagocytosis by a neutrophil or macrophage (Figure 3-4).

One important feature of the humoral immune system is that *each B-lymphocyte makes only one type of antibody,* with a single specificity for an antigen. Thus each B-lymphocyte is specific for one antigen.

HOW DOES THE IMMUNE SYSTEM RESPOND TO NEW AN-TIGENS? The number of different infectious agents and antigens that we might encounter during our lives is infinite. In order to protect us from disease, the immune system must be able to respond to each new antigen upon demand by making new antibodies that recognize it. On the other hand, it is impossible for the immune system to anticipate all possible antigens and continually make all possible antibodies that might be required all the time. This would be much too costly in terms of energy and genetic material. In order to solve this dilemma, the immune system uses two processes:

GENERATION OF ANTIBODY GENE DIVERSITY BY DNA REARRANGEMENT. The genetic information for the antibody proteins is contained within *DNA* in our chromosomes. DNA is a long molecule made up of two strands that are wound around each other. Each strand is a chain made up of building blocks called *nucleotides*, which contain four possible *bases* (adenine or A, cytosine or C, thymine or T and guanosine or G). The exact order of bases in a DNA molecule specifies the order of amino acid building blocks in the corresponding protein, as shown in Figure 3-9. The sequence of DNA bases that specifies one protein is referred to as a gene. Each of our chromosomes contains many thousands of genes along its DNA molecule. We inherit two sets of DNA molecules in the form of chromosomes — one set from our mother and one set from our father. The DNA content of most of the cells in the body is the same — different kinds of cells make different kinds of proteins by selecting which genes will be expressed by way of messenger RNA (see Chapter 4) synthesis into protein. However, antibody-producing B-lymphocytes are an exception, at least as far as the region of the chromosome that specifies antibody proteins is concerned.

It is important to remember that each mature B-lymphocyte only produces one kind of antibody. Thus each B-lymphocyte makes one kind of heavy chain protein, and one kind of light chain. All of the cells in the body actually contain multiple copies of the genes for variable regions of the heavy and light chain proteins. For the heavy chains, the variable region is actually expressed

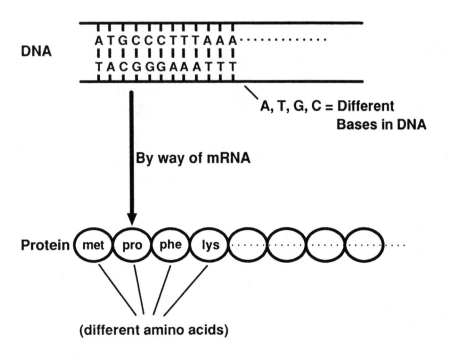

DNA

A, T, G, C = Different
Bases in DNA

By way of mRNA

Protein (met) (pro) (phe) (lys) · · · · · · · · · · · ·

(different amino acids)

FIGURE 3-9. How genetic information in DNA is converted into protein.

Before DNA Rearrangement

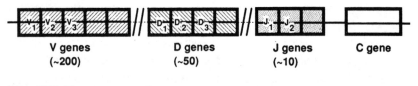

V genes (~200)   D genes (~50)   J genes (~10)   C gene

After DNA Rearrangement

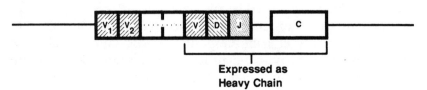

Expressed as
Heavy Chain

FIGURE 3-10. DNA rearrangement for expression of antibodies.

from three sets of genes called *V-genes, D-genes* and *J-genes*. There are about 200 different V-genes, about 50 different D-genes, and about ten different J-genes. During development and maturation of a B-lymphocyte, the DNA in the chromosomes surrounding the antibody genes is rearranged (Figure 3-10). As a result of the rearrangement, one V-gene is brought together with one D- and one J-gene, and this combination is next to the gene for the constant region. This VDJ combination is "expressed" along with the constant region gene to give the heavy chain protein. Light chain protein also results from a similar DNA rearrangement process, except that the variable region is specified by only two sets of multiple genes, V-genes and J-genes.

The DNA rearrangements of the antibody genes (VDJ for heavy chain and VJ for light chains) in any individual developing B-lymphocyte are *randomly selected* from the various possible V-, D- and J-genes. Thus the total number of possible VDJ combinations for the heavy chains in a B-lymphocyte is the *product* of the number of V-genes times the number of D-genes, times the number of J-genes (200 V-genes X 50 D-genes X 10 J-genes = 100,000 combinations for the variable region). Similarly, the total possible VJ combinations for light chain proteins is the product of the number of light chain V-genes times the number of light chain J-genes. Since each B-lymphocyte produces a unique kind of antibody containing one heavy chain and one light chain, the total number of possible antibodies a B-lymphocyte can make is the product of the possible kinds of heavy chain proteins times the possible kinds of light chain proteins. Thus the number of possible antibodies a B-lymphocyte can make is many millions.

Another process also takes place during B-lymphocyte maturation, in addition to the DNA rearrangement of the antibody genes. Individual DNA bases in the genes for the variable regions may be changed or added. These changes will further alter the amino acid sequences of the variable regions for the light and heavy chain proteins. Since these changes also occur on a random basis, they *further increase* the number of kinds of variable regions on the antibody proteins. In practice, the number of possible kinds of antibody proteins that can be made is almost limitless.

CLONAL SELECTION. In a normal, uninfected individual there are many different B-lymphocytes that have each carried out the DNA rearrangements of their antibody genes, and become more mature every day. Initially, these B-lymphocytes express their specific antibodies on their outer surfaces, but they do not secrete antibody and they do not divide. However, if a particular B-lymphocyte recognizes an antigen that binds to its specific antibody (for instance a protein from an infecting virus), it receives a *signal for activation*. Other B-lymphocytes that are present but that have not bound an antigen do not receive the activation signal. If the B-lymphocyte that has bound antigen also receives a *second signal* (see next page), it becomes *fully activated* (Figure 3-11). A fully activated B-lymphocyte does two things: 1) it *divides rapidly* and generates more activated B-cells that make the same antibody, and 2) these activated B-cells all *secrete the specific antibody* into the extracellular space (for instance the lymph or blood). The result of this process is the production of large amounts of antibody specific for the antigen.

THE PRIMARY IMMUNE RESPONSE occurs when the immune system encounters an antigen for the first time, as shown in Figure 3-12. For several days after an antigen is encountered, there are no antibodies for the antigen in the blood stream. This lag period can last for as little as ten days, or up to several weeks. During the lag period, B-lymphocytes are becoming primed with antigen, and being activated to divide and produce antibody. Eventually, antibodies specific for the antigen begin to appear in the blood stream, and increase until they reach a plateau level. Then, if the antigen is eliminated, the antibody level slowly falls until it returns to an undetectable (or barely detectable) level.

In terms of infectious agents such as viruses and bacteria, the lag period during the primary immune response is very important. During this period, no antibodies against the microorganism are being produced. Thus, the individual is susceptible to continued infection during this period — the immune system will begin to fight most efficiently only after antibodies are produced. This window of vulnerability is particularly critical for virus infections, since it is often very difficult to eliminate them once they have become established (see Chapter 4).

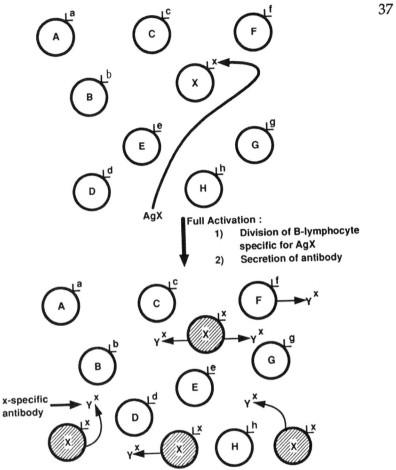

FIGURE 3-11. Clonal selection of B-lymphocytes.

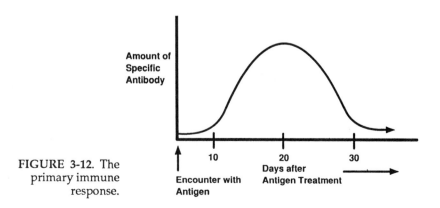

FIGURE 3-12. The primary immune response.

During the primary immune response, many different B-lymphocytes become primed and activated to produce antibodies. For instance, in the case of virus infections, B-lymphocytes that make antibodies specific for different virus proteins will be activated. Furthermore, different B-lymphocytes may make antibodies for different parts of a single virus protein. All of these B-lymphocytes contribute to the mixture of antibodies that makes up the immune response.

As the primary immune response progresses, the quality of the antibodies also improves. Those antibodies whose variable regions bind most tightly to the antigen become predominant. In addition, the nature of the constant regions of the antibody molecules change. This leads to more efficient signalling by the antibodies to other cells of the immune system (such as phagocytes) for attack and destruction of the foreign cell or microorganism.

A SECONDARY IMMUNE RESPONSE occurs in individuals who have previously raised an immunological reaction against a particular antigen, for instance someone who has recovered from an infection and then later encounters the same infectious agent. In this case, the levels of specific antibodies rise very rapidly, almost without a lag (Figure 3-13). The levels of specific antibody also fall more slowly than after the primary immune response. In addition, the antibodies are of the high quality kind, which bind antigen tightly and efficiently signal to other immune cells for attack. Thus the immune system is said to have *immunological memory* — the ability to respond rapidly and efficiently to an antigen that has been encountered previously.

The nature of the primary and secondary immune responses and immunological memory have led to development of *vaccines* and *vaccination* for controlling infections. The principle is to pre-expose an individual to part of an infectious agent, which cannot cause disease (the vaccine), and to induce production of antibodies against that agent. Repeated injections during the initial immunization are often used to induce the production of high quality antibodies. After the initial immunization, booster injections at regular intervals stimulate the immunological memory

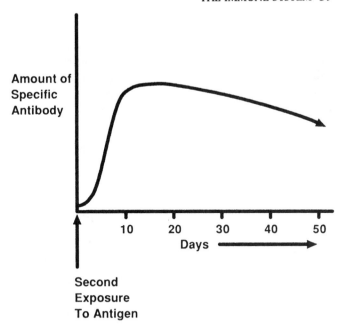

FIGURE 3-13. The secondary
immune response.

and maintain circulating antibodies for the infectious agent. These antibodies will prevent the infectious agent from getting established in a vaccinated individual.

Other tissues in our bodies contain many molecules that could possibly serve as antigens for our own immune systems. It would be very detrimental to our health if our immune systems attack our own tissues. Indeed, there are immunological disorders (for instance rheumatoid arthritis) called autoimmune diseases that consist of immunological attack by an individual's own tissue. In normal individuals the immune system distinguishes between *self* and *non-self*. This is achieved by the development of *tolerance* toward normal tissues. For the most part, this is accomplished by elimination during early development of B- and T-lymphocytes that recognize normal tissues. Since these "self"-specific lymphocytes are absent, no immunological response towards normal tissue will occur. In addition, there are other T-lymphocytes that provide a second line of defense should some "self"-specific lymphocytes avoid elimination. These lymphocytes are called $T_{suppressor}$ lymphocytes, and they prevent B-lymphocytes or T_{helper} lymphocytes specific for "self" antigens from maturing. $T_{suppressor}$ lymphocytes have CD8 protein on their surfaces, like T_{killer} lymphocytes.

A SUMMARY OF THE HUMORAL IMMUNE SYSTEM includes these points:

1) B-lymphocytes make antibody molecules, and each B-cell makes only one kind of antibody.

2) The immune response is based on a) generation of many B-lymphocytes with different antibody specificities by DNA rearrangement and mutation within the antibody genes, and b) clonal expansion of B-cells that recognize their specific antigen when infection occurs.

3) Antibodies fight infections by a) direct neutralization of viruses, b) binding to targets and signaling phagocytes or other white blood cells to attack, or c) binding to target cells and signaling for other host defense mechanisms.

T-CELLS AND CELL-MEDIATED IMMUNITY. As described above, T-cells make *T-cell antigen receptors* that resemble antibodies made by B-cells. As with an antibody, the T-cell receptor variable region determines its specificity toward an antigen. Also like B-lymphocytes, each T-lymphocyte makes only one kind of T-cell antigen receptor. Thus, each T-lymphocyte is specific for a particular antigen. As described previously, T-lymphocytes do not release their receptors; instead, the receptors are anchored in the cell surface with the variable regions projecting outside. As a result, T-lymphocytes will bind to cells expressing antigen by way of their T-cell antigen receptor. T-lymphocytes represent *cell-mediated immunity*, since the cells themselves specifically bind with antigens. This contrasts with humoral immunity in which antibodies released from B-lymphocytes carry out the antigen binding.

T$_{\text{KILLER}}$ LYMPHOCYTES bind cells carrying a foreign antigen and directly kill those cells. Once they have carried out this killing, they release from the target cell, which has been destroyed, and can bind and kill other cells. An example of such an interaction is shown in Figure 3-14. Some examples of cells that T$_{\text{killer}}$ cells attack include:

1) *Virus-infected cells.* Most cells infected with viruses express some of the viral proteins on their outer surfaces. These viral proteins can be recognized as foreign antigens and bind T$_{\text{killer}}$ lymphocytes. As a result, the virus-infected cells will be killed.

T$_{\text{k}}$ Target Cell

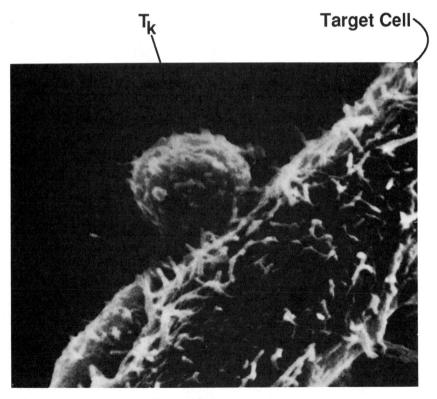

FIGURE 3-14.
T$_{\text{killer}}$ lymphocyte killing a target cell (electron microscope picture).

2) *Tumor cells.* When cancers develop, they often express abnormal proteins on their outer surfaces. These abnormal proteins can also provoke an immune response by T-lymphocytes, which results in immunological attack of the tumor cells. In fact, the immune system is an important part of our natural defense against cancer. During our lives probably many cells in our bodies begin to develop into tumors, but the cell-mediated immune system eliminates them before they can grow very much. This is called *immunological surveillance.* This is also important in AIDS, because as we shall see, failure of the immune system can result in development of cancers. In addition to T-lymphocytes, natural killer cells are also very important in immunological surveillance.

3) *Tissue Rejection.* When tissue from an unrelated individual is introduced into another person, the cell-mediated immune system will generally raise a strong response and kill the transplanted tissue. This is because cell surface proteins called *histocompatability antigens* generally differ from individual to individual. This is a major problem for medical procedures such as skin grafting and organ transplantation. If tissue with different histocompatibility antigens is transplanted into an individual, a strong cell-mediated immune response against these antigens will occur and the transplanted tissue will be destroyed. In the case of organ transplantation donors and recipients must be carefully matched for histocompatibility antigens, in order to avoid rejection of the donor organ.

THELPER LYMPHOCYTES play a central role in both humoral and cell-mediated immunity. In *humoral immunity* they provide the second signal necessary for a B-lymphocyte that has bound antigen to divide and secrete antibodies (Figure 3-11). In fact, in order for a B-lymphocyte that has bound antigen to become fully activated, a Thelper lymphocyte with the *same antigenic specificity*

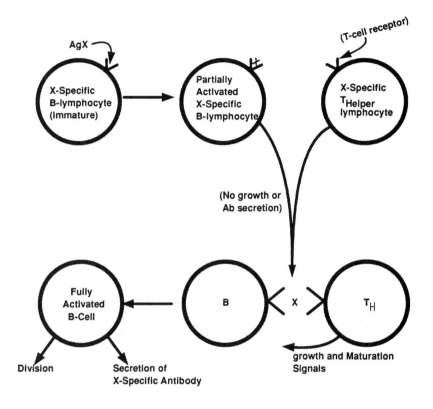

FIGURE 3-15. T_{helper} cells and B-lymphocyte activation.

must bind the antigen as well, as shown in Figure 3-15. Once the specific T_{helper} lymphocyte is bound to the B-lymphocyte by way of the antigen, it provides growth and maturation signals to the B-cell leading to growth and antibody production. It is important that if a T_{helper} lymphocyte of the same antigen specificity as the B-lymphocyte is absent, the B-lymphocyte will not complete maturation, even if it has bound antigen.

T_{helper} cells also play an important role in *cell-mediated* immunity. When T-lymphocytes (either T_{helper} or T_{killer}) bind antigen, they become activated to divide. This will result in increased numbers of specific T-lymphocytes to fight the foreign infectious agent. However, as with many blood cells, T-lympho-

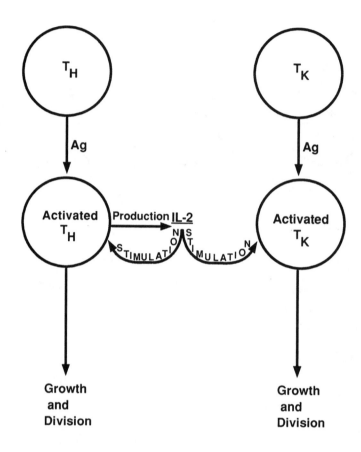

FIGURE 3-16. T$_{helper}$ cells in cell-mediated immunity.

cytes also need a growth factor in order to divide. For T-lymphocytes that have bound antigen, the required growth factor is one
called interleukin 2 or IL-2. It turns out that T$_{helper}$ lymphocytes
produce and secrete IL-2 when they are activated by antigen
binding (Figure 3-16). Thus the T$_{helper}$ lymphocytes can stimulate themselves to divide after they bind antigen. On the other
hand, most T$_{killer}$ cells do not produce IL-2 even after they bind
antigen. They generally rely on IL-2 secreted by neighboring
T$_{helper}$ cells in order to divide. In this case, the neighboring

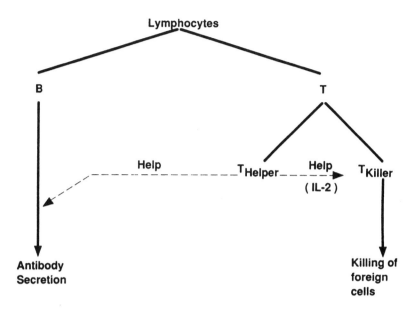

FIGURE 3-17. The central role of T_{helper} lymphocytes.

T_{helper} cell that produces the IL-2 does not have to be specific for the same antigen as the T_{killer} cell that it helps. Thus, if T_{helper} lymphocytes are absent, T_{killer} cells cannot divide even if they have bound their specific antigens.

In summary, T_{helper} lymphocytes play a central role in both humoral and cell-mediated immunity, as illustrated in Figure 3-17. As we shall see in the next chapter, the major problem in AIDS is that the causative agent HIV specifically infects and kills T_{helper} lymphocytes. This will cause a failure of both the humoral immune system and in cell-mediated immunity. As a result, there will be little immunological protection against infectious agents or development of cancer.

4

VIROLOGY AND HUMAN IMMUNODEFICIENCY VIRUS

I N THIS CHAPTER we shall first look at viruses in general, then retoviruses, and then HIV, the virus that causes AIDS in particular. We will also see how the HIV antibody test (used to screen for HIV infection) works, and what it tells us. We will then consider the basis of action of the drug azidothymidine (AZT), which is currently the approved anti-viral treatment for HIV infection.

A GENERAL INTRODUCTION TO VIRUSES

Let's first consider viruses in a general sense. There are many different kinds of viruses that cause many diseases. Individual viruses may differ in their exact compositions and mechanisms for growth, but all viruses have some properties in common.

WHAT ARE VIRUSES? Viruses are the simplest microorganisms that exist. Here are some of the common features of viruses:

1) *Viruses are obligate intracellular parasites.* This means that viruses cannot replicate and make more of themselves outside of cells. In fact, a pure preparation of virus particles will not grow. In the case of humans, this means that viruses must replicate in some tissue or cell type in our bodies.

2) *Virus particles consist of* (see Figure 4-1):

a) *Genetic material.* Viruses carry genetic material in the form of *nucleic acids.* For some viruses the nucleic acid is *DNA,* the same as the genetic material of the cells in our body. For other viruses the nucleic acid is *RNA,* which is related chemically to DNA — more about this later. *The genetic material of a virus specifies virus proteins.* These virus proteins may be *structural proteins* that make up the virus particles, *enzymes* that help carry out biochemical processes necessary for virus growth, or they may be *regulatory proteins.* Some viral regulatory proteins are used by the virus to select expression of particular virus genes at different times or under different conditions. Other viral regulatory proteins may be used by the virus to help take over the cell and convert it into an efficient "factory" for producing virus.

b) *A system for protecting the genetic material and introducing it into a cell.* Viruses must protect their genetic material when they leave one cell and move to another — either within tissues of an infected individual, or from an infected individual to an uninfected one. Naked DNA or RNA is quite fragile and vulnerable to attack by numerous agents. Thus, viruses carry genes that direct production of a *protein coat* that surrounds the genetic material. In addition, some (but not all) viruses also direct

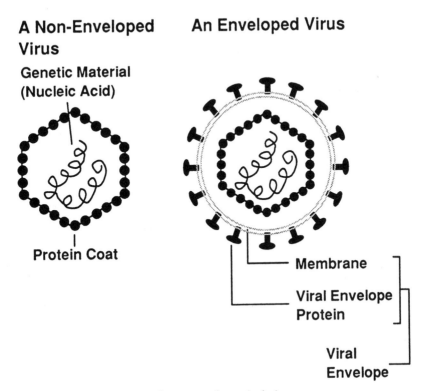

FIGURE 4-1. Structure of a typical virus.

synthesis of a *viral envelope* that surrounds the virus genetic information and protein coat. Viral envelopes resemble the membranes that make up the outer surfaces of our cells. These membranes contain proteins that are virus-specified. For viruses that contain envelopes, the envelope proteins are very important for the initial phases of infection, since they are exposed on the outside of the virus particle.

3) *Viruses are dependent on cells for:*

a) *Energy metabolism.* Energy is required for most biochemical processes to take place. In the case of viruses, such processes include those responsible for production of the virus proteins and genetic material. However, viruses themselves do not carry the machinery necessary for generating energy. Instead, they rely upon the machinery of the cell they infect.

b) *Protein synthesis.* Proteins are synthesized in cells by a complex system of molecules and sub-cellular particles, using instructions from the genetic material. Again, viruses carry the genetic instructions but do not carry the machinery for synthesis of proteins. They depend upon the cell protein synthesis machinery.

c) *Nucleic acid synthesis.* Many viruses may also depend on the cell machinery for synthesis of virus-specific nucleic acids. These nucleic acids may be used for expression of viral proteins (mRNA) or they may be the virus genetic information itself.

HOW DOES A VIRUS INFECT A HOST? In order for a virus to infect an individual, it must come into contact with a susceptible cell. It is important to remember that most of our body is covered with skin, which is designed to protect us from infection: skin is quite tough, and the outer layers of skin cells are actually dead. Thus most viruses cannot infect and grow in cells of the outer layers of the skin. These are some of the important routes into the body that viruses use (Figure 4-2):

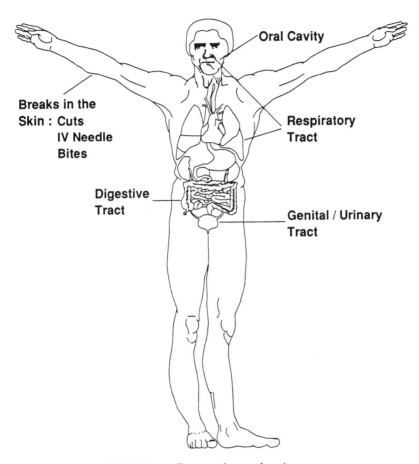

FIGURE 4-2. Routes of entry for viruses.

1) *The respiratory tract.* Viruses can be carried into the respiratory tract through the air that we breathe. Once they are brought into the body by this route, they can infect cells in any part of the respiratory tract, including the nose, wind pipe, bronchial tubes and lungs. Examples of viruses that infect the respiratory tract are influenza and the common cold.

2) *The oral cavity and digestive tract.* If viruses are taken in with food or water, they can potentially infect cells of the mouth and other parts of the digestive system, includ-

ing the large and small intestines. The virus that causes one form of liver inflammation or hepatitis ("infectious" or type A hepatitis) is an example of this category, as are viruses that cause various diarrheas.

3) *The genital tract.* During sexual intercourse it is possible to introduce viruses into the female or male genital tract from an infected partner. Such infections are classified as venereal diseases. If sexual intercourse involves anal penetration, it is also possible to introduce viruses into the anus, rectum and lower intestines by this route as well. Genital herpes virus is an example of an infection of the genital tract. As we shall see, genital tract infection is an important route for HIV and AIDS.

4) *Breaks in the skin.* If the protective layer of skin is broken by a cut or scratch, then viruses may be able to enter directly into tissues or the blood stream. *Bites from animals or insects* also fall into this category. For example, rabies is spread by bites from infected animals such as dogs or squirrels, and yellow fever is spread by bites from infected mosquitoes. *Transfusions* and *IV drug abuse* are other examples of this category. In these cases, viruses that contaminate blood or blood products can be introduced into individuals during intravenous transfusions with blood or blood products, or during intravenous drug abuse involving shared needles. An example of this is the virus that causes another form of hepatitis, hepatitis B. IV drug abuse (and originally transfusions) is another important route of infection for HIV.

It is important to remember that any individual type of virus will use some but not all of these routes of infection. A key to controlling a viral infection is understanding the particular routes of spread that the virus uses. We shall see how this is determined in Chapter 6. Once a virus has entered an individual and established infection at a *primary site*, the infection can spread to *secondary sites* in the body as well. Disease symptoms may result from infection at the primary site, the secondary sites, or both.

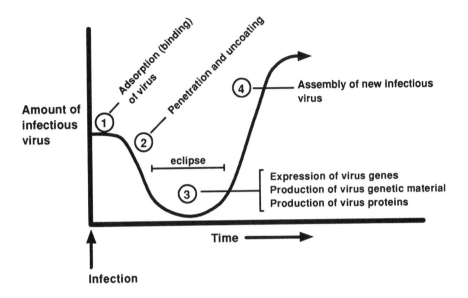

FIGURE 4-3. A typical virus infection cycle.

A TYPICAL VIRUS INFECTION CYCLE. Let's look at what happens if a purified virus preparation is used to infect some susceptible cells in the laboratory. A typical result is shown in Figure 4-3. If the amount of infectious virus is measured over a period of time, it is seen to fall after an initial lag period, remain low for a period of time, and then rise to even higher levels. The period during which the amount of infectious virus is low is referred to as the *eclipse* period. The virus infection cycle can be divided into several events:

1) *Adsorption (binding)* of the virus to the cell. When a virus infects, it must first bind to the cell. This binding is a very specific interaction between the virus particle and some protein (or other molecule) on the cell surface. This protein is referred to as the virus *receptor*. At first it might seem strange that cells have receptors for viruses,

since this would seem to be disadvantageous to the uninfected host. However, this is due to the fact that viruses have evolved so that they are able to bind to a protein that is normally present on the uninfected cell. The distribution of the receptor protein among different cells in the body will influence the kinds of cells that the virus can infect. We will see that this is an important consideration for HIV infection and development of AIDS.

2) *Penetration* of the virus into the cell and *uncoating* of the viral genetic material. Once the virus particles have bound to the surface of the cell by attaching to a receptor protein, they are brought into the cell. This penetration process is an active one, which requires expenditure of energy by the cell. Once the virus particle has been taken into the cell, the protective protein coat is removed, exposing the viral genetic material. The genetic material is now ready to be expressed. This uncoating of the virus accounts for the drop in infectious virus assayed because the uncoated virus cannot withstand the assay conditions.

3) *Expression of the viral genetic material.* This occurs during the eclipse period, when the amount of infectious virus in the culture appears low. Several events take place during the eclipse phase:

a) *Organization of the infected cell for virus expression.* The cell machinery may be altered to favor efficient expression of virus genes. This often occurs at expense of the cell's own metabolic processes, and may ultimately lead to death of the infected cell.

b) *Replication of the viral genetic material.* The virus programs the machinery necessary to generate more copies of its own genetic material. In some cases, this may rely on machinery from the uninfected cell, but in other cases, the virus may specify proteins that are necessary for the process.

c) *Synthesis of proteins for virus particles.* Proteins that make up the virus coat, as well as those in the viral envelope, are synthesized from instructions in the viral genetic information. Once these proteins are synthesized, all of the components necessary for formation of a new virus particle are present within the infected cell.

4) *Assembly of virus particles and release* from the cell. Virus particles are assembled in the infected cell from the new genetic material and viral proteins. As this occurs, the amount of infectious virus in the culture will increase and surpass that at the start of the infection. Typically, an infected cell will release hundreds or thousands of new virus particles that can spread to infect other cells.

Depending on the virus, there are different fates for an infected cell. For many viruses the infected cell is killed (or lysed) at the end of the infection. These viruses are called *lytic*. Other viruses do not kill the infected cell, but they establish a persistent or carrier state where the cell survives and continually produces virus particles. These viruses are called *non-lytic*. Some viruses can also establish a state called *latency* in cells. In these situations, the virus genetic material remains hidden in the cell, but no virus is produced. At a later time, the latent virus can become *reactivated*, and the cell will begin to produce infectious virus particles again, as in the case of cold sores caused by a herpes virus. As we shall see, all of these fates probably play an important role in HIV infection and the development of AIDS.

HOW DO WE TREAT VIRAL INFECTIONS? Once virus infections become established, they are very difficult to treat. This contrasts with the wide variety of antibiotics that are available to treat infections by other microorganisms such as bacteria and fungi. Antibiotics take advantage of the fact that there are differences in some of the biochemical machinery of these very simple microorganisms compared to highly developed organisms such as humans. These antibiotics specifically inhibit processes carried out by the bacteria or fungi, but they do not affect similar processes in higher organisms. For instance, the antibiotic streptomycin inhibits the machinery used to make proteins in bacteria, but not in humans. Unfortunately, since viruses rely on the cell to carry out most of their metabolic processes, it is difficult to find drugs similar to classical antibiotics that will block virus growth without killing the infected cell. However, in a few cases, compounds that specifically inhibit a viral process have been identified. These compounds are called *anti-virals*, and they hold the key for future treatment of viral infections. As we shall see, there is one anti-viral that inhibits HIV infection to some degree and slows up the progress of AIDS, azidothymidine (zidovudine or AZT). At the present time, the basic treatment for most virus infections is to manage the symptoms and wait for the infection to run its course. Management of symptoms can include treatment to reduce fevers (for instance aspirin), classical antibiotics (to prevent secondary infections by bacteria in a weakened individual), and bed rest.

Since treatment of virus infections is currently not very effective, the best approach to managing viral disease is to prevent the initial infection. One powerful method is public health and sanitation methods to intervene in the epidemiological cycle of the virus, as described in Chapter 2. Another important approach is the use of viral *vaccines*, as described in Chapter 3. If immunity to a virus can be induced by the vaccine before a person encounters the virus, then it will not be able to establish a foothold. Most of you are probably familiar with some of the best-known virus vaccines, which include the smallpox vaccine developed by Edward Jenner (the first vaccine), rabies vaccine developed by Louis Pasteur, and polio vaccines developed by Jonas Salk and Albert Sabin.

THE LIFE CYCLE OF A RETROVIRUS

HIV belongs to a class of viruses called retroviruses. Let's examine the life cycle of a typical retrovirus.

Before considering the retrovirus life cycle, it is important to discuss the *central dogma for genetic information flow* in cells. The central dogma states that genetic information flows in this direction:

DNA —> RNA —> Protein

That is, the genetic information is carried in *DNA* as a sequence of nucleotide bases (see Figure 3-9, Chapter 3). In higher organisms the DNA is organized into chromosomes that are located in the *nucleus* of the cell. When a gene is "expressed," the information from the DNA base sequence is copied or transferred (transcribed) to a related molecule called *RNA* using the DNA molecule as a pattern. The RNA (which is called *messenger RNA* or *mRNA*) then moves from the cell nucleus to the *cytoplasm*. Once in the cytoplasm, the messenger RNA is used as a blueprint for the formation of *proteins* (translation). The proteins then carry out most of the important functions for the cell.

The structure of a retrovirus is shown in Figure 4-4. The genetic information of a retrovirus is *RNA*. This RNA is covered with a viral *protein coat*; together the viral RNA and coat protein make up a *core* particle. The core particle also contains several virus-specified enzymes. The core particle is surrounded by a viral *envelope*, which contains membrane lipids and viral envelope protein.

The life cycle of a retrovirus is shown in Figure 4-5. The retrovirus first binds to the surface of an uninfected cell by recognizing a cell receptor. After binding, the virus particle is brought into the cytoplasm of the cell. During this process the viral envelope is removed, leaving the core particle. Once this happens, a unique virus-specified enzyme in the core particle called *reverse transcriptase* is activated. This enzyme reads the viral RNA and *makes viral DNA*. The host cell lacks such an enzyme. The viral DNA then moves to the nucleus of the cell, where it is incorporated (or *integrated*) into the host cell's DNA in the chromosomes. Once this viral DNA is integrated into the chromosome, it resembles any other cell gene. As a result, the normal cell machinery reads the integrated viral DNA to make more copies of viral RNA. This viral RNA is then used for *two purposes*: 1) some of the viral RNA moves to the cytoplasm and functions as *viral messenger RNA* to program

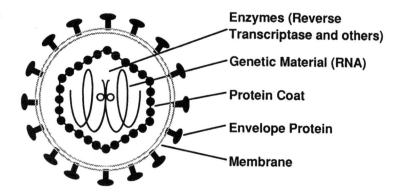

The RNA Genetic Material

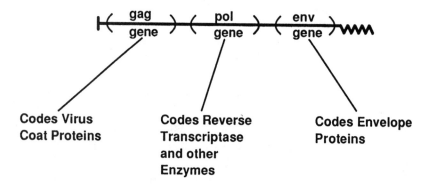

FIGURE 4-4. The structure of a retrovirus.

the formation of *viral proteins;* 2) the rest of the viral RNA becomes *genetic material* for new virus particles by moving to the cytoplasm and combining with viral proteins. These virus particles are formed at the cell surface and leave the cell by a process called *budding.*

There are several important characteristics of the retrovirus life cycle. First, most retroviruses do not kill the cell that they infect. Second, the fact that these viruses integrate their DNA into

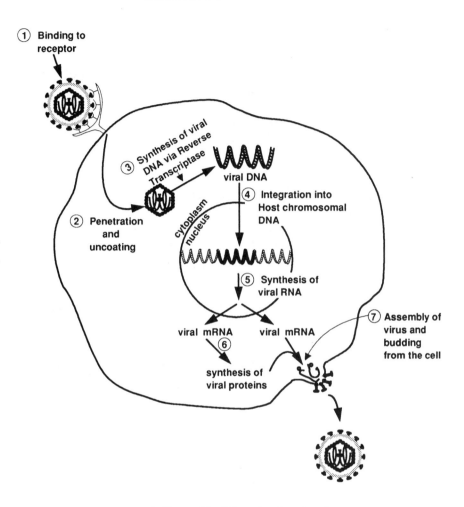

FIGURE 4-5. The life cycle of a retrovirus.

host chromosomes means that they establish a stable carrier state within the infected cell. As a result, once cells are infected with most retroviruses, they will continually produce virus without dying. For some retroviruses, a latent state may also be established, in which the retroviral DNA is integrated into the host chromosomes, but it does not program formation of new virus particles. However, at a later time (sometimes years later), the latent viral DNA may become activated by some means, and virus will be produced. This latency process is probably important in AIDS. The viral enzyme reverse transcriptase carries out an unusual process in converting the viral RNA genetic information into DNA. This is the *reverse* of genetic information flow according to the central dogma of molecular biology. This is the reason the enzyme is called reverse transcriptase. This is also where retroviruses get their name — "retro" is from the Latin word for reverse.

In terms of their genetic material, all retroviruses have three genes (see Figure 4-4). These genes code for:

1) *Coat proteins that make up the inner virus (core) particle.* The virus gene that specifies these proteins is called the *gag* gene. For HIV, there are three *gag* proteins, called p17, p24, and p15.

2) *The enzyme reverse transcriptase, as well as some other enzymes used in virus replication.* The gene that codes these enzymes is the *pol* gene.

3) *The proteins of the viral envelope.* The gene that codes for these proteins is the *env* gene. A protein coded by the *env* gene is responsible for binding of the virus to the cell receptor. For HIV, there are two *env* proteins, gp120 and gp41.

THE AIDS VIRUS: HIV

The virus that causes AIDS is Human Immunodeficiency Virus (HIV) (Figure 4-6). Other names that have been used previously for HIV include HTLV-III, LAV and ARV. HIV belongs to a subgroup of retroviruses called *lentiviruses* (meaning "slow" viruses, since they often cause disease extremely slowly); other lentiviruses have been found in such diverse species as cats, sheep, goats, horses and monkeys. Actually, the virus responsible for the great majority of AIDS cases in the United States, Europe and Africa is called HIV-1. Recently, a second virus related to HIV-1 has been isolated in Africa, HIV-2 (see Chapter 6). HIV-2 also appears to

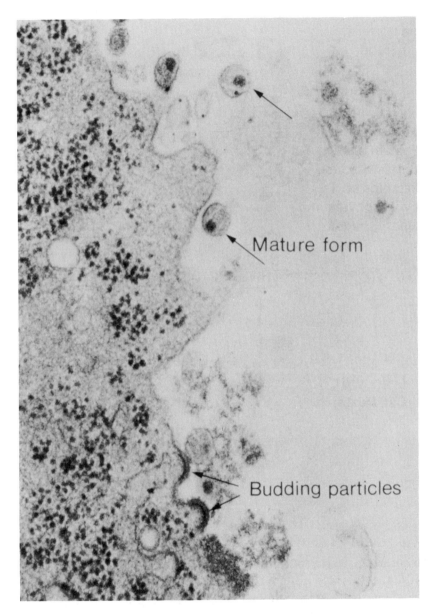

FIGURE 4-6. An electron miscroscope picture of an HIV-infected cell. The cytoplasm of the cell is on the left, and the exterior of the cell is on the right. Budding HIV particles are indicated, as well as mature virus particles released from the cell. (*Courtesy of the Center for Disease Control*)

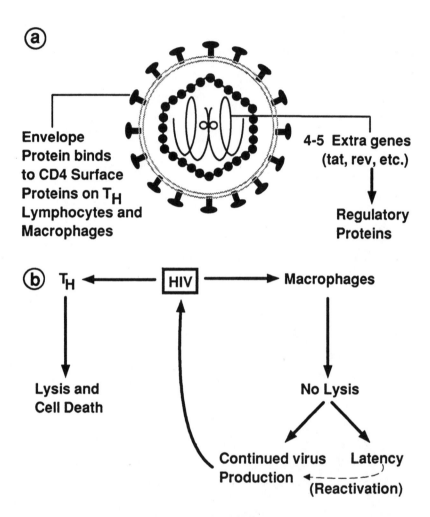

FIGURE 4-7. Unusual features of HIV.

cause AIDS. In this book we will refer to the AIDS virus simply as HIV, and this will almost always mean HIV-1.

Several features about the structure or replication of HIV are important, as shown in Figure 4-7a:

1) *The nature of the HIV receptor.* The cell receptor that HIV binds to is the *CD4 surface protein.* As described in

Chapter 2, CD4 protein is present on Thelper lymphocytes. In fact, this is the predominant cell type that has CD4 protein. In addition, some macrophages also have CD4 protein as well. Most other cells in the body do *not* contain CD4 protein. As a result, *the main cells that HIV can infect are Thelper lymphocytes and macrophages.* The HIV envelope protein responsible for virus binding to CD4 protein is called gp120.

2) *Extra genes.* As for all retroviruses, HIV contains the three genes for coat proteins, reverse transcriptase, and envelope proteins (*gag, pol* and *env*). In addition, HIV contains genes that specify six additional proteins. These proteins are regulatory proteins that give HIV finer levels of control and a more versatile life cycle. Two of the best known of these genes are:

> *tat,* which is an up-regulator or amplifier of viral gene expression in the infected cell, and

> *rev,* which shifts the balance from production of viral regulatory proteins to proteins that make up virus particles.

These extra genes may be important in allowing the virus to establish a latent or inactive state in some infected cells, followed by reactivation at later times.

3) *Killing of Thelper lymphocytes.* In contrast to most retroviral infections, *infection of Thelper lymphocytes with HIV results in cell death* (Figure 4-7b). Considering the pivotal role that Thelper lymphocytes play in both humoral and cell-mediated immunity (see Chapter 3), it is possible to understand how infection with HIV can ultimately lead to collapse of the immune system.

4) *Non-lytic infection of macrophages.* When HIV infects macrophages, it follows a course that is typical of other retroviruses, in that the infected macrophages are not killed (Figure 4-7b). In most cases, the macrophages continue to produce HIV virus particles, while other macrophages establish a latent state of HIV infection. These infected macrophages are an important reservoir

of infection in an HIV-infected individual. This may also explain how many years can elapse between the time of initial infection and development of clinical AIDS symptoms.

THE EFFECTS OF HIV INFECTION IN INDIVIDUALS. Let's now consider the results of HIV infection at the level of infected people. As the routes of HIV infection will be covered in Chapters 6 and 7, we will start here at the time a person becomes infected. There will be a detailed description of AIDS as a clinical disease in the next chapter, but an overview is useful at this point.

The progression of events after HIV infection is shown in Figure 4-8. After HIV infection, there are generally very few initial symptoms — perhaps a mild flu-like illness or swollen glands. Most individuals then remain free of any clinical symptoms for variable lengths of time — up to many years. Individuals who are HIV-infected but who do not show any signs of disease are referred to as *asymptomatic*. It is generally difficult to detect infectious HIV virus in infected asymptomatic individuals. Indeed,

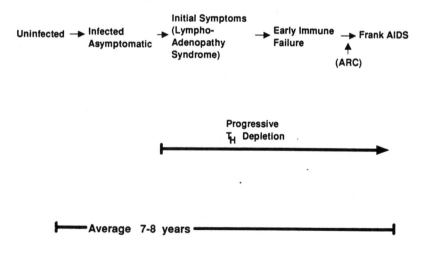

FIGURE 4-8. Consequences of HIV infection.

even as individuals develop signs of clinical symptoms, they generally have rather low levels of infectious HIV. One of the puzzles about HIV is how it can cause such devastating disease with such apparently low levels of circulating virus. During the asymptomatic period, individuals generally produce *antibodies* to HIV. Unfortunately, these antibodies are not sufficient to prevent continued HIV infection as the disease progresses. However, they provide a useful diagnosis for HIV infection, as we shall see in the following pages.

As time passes, many HIV-infected individuals begin to experience symptoms of HIV infection. Some initial symptoms include persistent enlarged lymph glands (*lymphadenopathy syndrome* or *LAS*), and fevers or night-sweats. As the disease worsens, a continuum of progressively more serious conditions develop as the immune system weakens, ultimately resulting in full-blown or Frank AIDS. During the early periods of the AIDS epidemic, doctors also used a classification called ARC or AIDS-related Complex. Individuals were classified as having ARC if they showed fewer of the characteristic opportunistic infections or cancers than patients with Frank AIDS. The term ARC is used less frequently today after the progressive nature of HIV infection has become apparent. The progression from asymptomatic infection to AIDS is accompanied by a progressive depletion of Thelper lymphocytes by HIV infection. Ultimately, there is a profound lack of Thelper lymphocytes, which results in the failure of both humoral and cell-mediated immunity.

The clinical manifestations of AIDS will be covered in detail in Chapter 5. They can be summarized briefly here:

1) *Opportunistic infections.* These are infections by microorganisms that normally do not cause problems in healthy individuals. However, in individuals with weakened immune systems, these microorganisms can take hold and cause devastating infections. One important opportunistic infection is a pneumonia caused by a fungus microbe called *pneumocystis carinii* (*PCP pneumonia*).

2) *Cancers.* Cell-mediated immunity also plays an important role in defense against development of cancers (immune surveillance — see Chapter 3). HIV-infected individuals develop several cancers with very high frequency. One example of an AIDS-related cancer is *Kaposi's sarcoma.*

3) *Weight loss.* Many AIDS patients suffer from profound weight loss or wasting. The mechanism for this is not yet understood .

4) *Mental impairment.* HIV can also establish infection in the nervous system. This can result in muscle spasms or tics. More serious, infection of the central nervous system can result in *AIDS-related dementia* in which individuals lose the ability to reason.

Individual AIDS patients may suffer from one or more of these manifestations. Indeed, recurrent bouts with different opportunistic infections or cancers may be experienced.

Since the major problem in AIDS is a loss of T_{helper} lymphocyte function, monitoring of the numbers of T_{helper} lymphocytes is important in clinical treatment of HIV-infected individuals. Doctors can perform a test for these cells, and the results are reported in terms of T_{helper} (or T4 or CD4) lymphocyte numbers. A few years ago the tests were frequently reported as the ratio of T_{helper} to T_{killer} lymphocytes in the blood (also T4/T8 or helper-to-suppressor ratios). An inversion of the normal T_{helper}/T_{killer} lymphocyte ratio is often an early sign of HIV infection.

The likelihood that an HIV-infected individual will develop full-blown AIDS will be discussed in more detail in Chapter 6. Current estimates are that more than 70% of HIV-infected individuals will develop AIDS with an average time to disease of eight or more years.

THE HIV ANTIBODY TEST. Within a year of the isolation of HIV as the causative agent of AIDS, a test was developed that determines if an individual has been exposed to HIV. The procedure is to test whether an individual has antibodies to HIV virus proteins. These

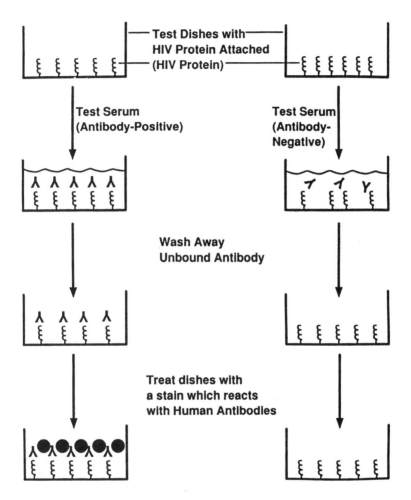

FIGURE 4-9. The ELISA test for HIV antibody.

antibodies appear in those who have been previously infected with HIV and made antibodies against the virus (see Chapter 3).

The most common HIV antibody test is called an *ELISA* test, shown in Figure 4-9. In an ELISA assay, virus protein is first attached to a small laboratory dish. A serum sample is prepared from the blood of the individual to be tested, and placed in the dish containing bound HIV viral proteins. If HIV-specific antibodies

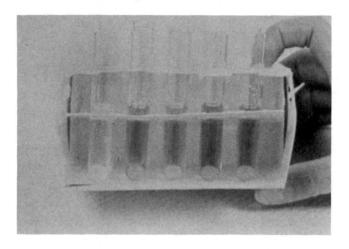

FIGURE 4-10. A modified ELISA test is shown. In this case, the virus proteins are attached to small beads that can float in solution, instead of the bottom of the dish. The tube on the left shows a test of a blood sample that does not have HIV-specific antibodies. The four tubes on the right show test of HIV antibody-positive blood samples. The color in the tubes on the right indicates the presence of HIV antibodies. (*Courtesy of Abbot Laboratories, Diagnostic Division*)

are present in the serum, they will become tightly bound to the dish by way of the HIV proteins. The serum is then removed and the dish is washed — during this procedure, only antibodies specific for HIV will be retained. The dish is then reacted with a stain that will detect *any* human antibodies. Thus, dishes that were exposed to serum containing HIV-specific antibodies will be stained, while dishes from antibody-negative serum samples will be unstained. This procedure has been automated, so that many blood samples can be tested at once (see Figure 4-10 for a variation of this). The current ELISA tests are better than 99.9% accurate. That is, less than 0.1% of HIV-negative individuals (one in a thousand) incorrectly score as positive by the ELISA test. Likewise, less than 0.1% of HIV antibody-positive serum samples are missed by the test.

POTENTIAL PROBLEMS WITH THE HIV ANTIBODY TEST.
Although this test has been extremely important in furthering our
knowledge of how the virus spreads and causes disease, there are
several potential problems as well:

1) *False positives.* These are individuals who are not HIV-
   infected, but who test antibody-positive in the ELISA
   assay. Clearly this can be an extremely frightening
   experience. With current ELISA assays, the frequency
   of false positives is less than one in one thousand (0.1%)
   uninfected individuals. False positives are a particular
   problem if populations with low frequencies of HIV
   infection are tested. In these cases, a high proportion of
   the individuals who score positive could be false positives. This is one of the arguments (besides cost) against
   routine HIV antibody screening of the general U.S.
   population, where current prevalences of infection are
   less than 1% — many of the individuals identified as
   antibody-positive in such a mass screening could be
   false positives.

   Because of the significant false positive rate for the
   ELISA test, a second more specific test for HIV antibodies is also used, the *Western blot* test. This technique
   has a lower incidence of false positives than the ELISA
   assay. In practice, serum samples that score antibody-
   positive by the ELISA test are generally re-tested by the
   Western blot procedure. Serum samples are considered
   positive if they are found to contain HIV-specific antibodies by both tests. New and improved tests (more
   sensitive and/or more accurate) for HIV infection are
   currently undergoing development.

2) *False negatives.* An equally important problem is individuals infected with HIV but who do not score positive
   in the HIV antibody test. Such individuals fall into two
   categories:

   a) *Recently infected individuals.* As was discussed in
   Chapter 3, the immune system has a lag period between

initial exposure to an antigen and the production of antibodies. In the case of HIV infection, this lag can range up to six months. Thus individuals who have been recently infected with HIV will not score positive in the antibody test.

b) *Infected individuals who never mount an immune response.* Since the immune response varies from person to person, a few infected individuals do not produce antibodies to HIV. There are rare but documented cases of individuals who remain antibody-negative but spread HIV infection to their sexual partners.

The HIV antibody test measures whether an individual has circulating antibodies to HIV. However, strictly speaking the test does *not* indicate if an antibody-positive individual still harbors infectious virus. Some individuals who are exposed to HIV might have raised a successful immune response and completely eliminated the infection. However, by and large, most HIV-antibody positive individuals turn out to be still infected.

While the HIV antibody test is the routine test used to identify individuals who have been exposed to HIV, other tests for viral infection are used as well. In particular, it is advantageous to know the amount of circulating virus particles in an infected individual, since the levels of virus are generally low, but they frequently rise when Frank AIDS develops. The most common test for virus particles is to measure the level of the major HIV core protein (p24 protein) in the blood. Because this test detects p24 protein by use of an antibody against it, it is sometimes referred to as a test for p24 antigen.

More sensitive tests for HIV infection are under development. This is important, because in an HIV-infected individual most cells are not infected — even among CD4-positive T$_{Helper}$ lymphocytes and monocytes/macrophages. A newly developed technique called *polymerase chain reaction* or PCR has been developed that tests for HIV DNA in infected cells. The PCR test can detect as few as one HIV-infected cell among a million uninfected ones, and is currently being used in research laboratories.

HOW DOES HIV EVADE THE IMMUNE SYSTEM? One of the paradoxes about HIV infection is that most infected individuals contain HIV antibodies, but the disease eventually occurs in most cases, even in the presence of these antibodies. This means that HIV antibodies are unable to prevent onset of AIDS. This may be due to several factors. First, the levels of antibodies raised might be insufficient to block spread of infectious virus. In addition, antibodies can be produced against different parts of the virus. Only some of these antibodies (*neutralizing antibodies*) can inactivate virus and prevent infection. Finally, several unique features of HIV infection provide the virus with ways to evade the immune system. These include:

1) *High mutation rates* for genes coding for the HIV envelope protein. The HIV envelope proteins are on the outside of the virus particle, and they are important in attaching the virus to the cell receptor. As such, they are the most important targets for neutralizing antibodies. However, HIV shows an unusually high mutation rate for its *env* gene, so that the exact amino acid sequence of the envelope proteins changes quite rapidly during successive cycles of infection. Changes in the makeup of HIV envelope proteins have even been observed over time within the same person. Thus, even though an infected individual may raise neutralizing antibodies to the initial infecting virus, those antibodies may not be able to neutralize subsequent viruses with mutated envelope proteins. Thus HIV can keep one step ahead of the immune system and continue infection.

2) HIV can establish *latent states* in some cells. In these cells, the viral DNA is maintained, but virus proteins are not expressed. As a result, these latently infected cells will not be recognized or attacked by the immune system, but remain as reservoirs for infectious virus. At later times, the virus may be activated from these cells. Macrophages are probably the major cells that carry latent HIV, since initial HIV infection does not kill them.

In addition, T$_{helper}$ cells latently infected with HIV may also exist, although in fewer numbers than latently infected macrophages.

Reactivation of latent HIV from carrier cells may also be important in AIDS progression. Infection of cells carrying latent HIV with certain other viruses, such as herpes simplex or cytomegalovirus, may reactivate the HIV. In addition, other stimuli to the immune system (such as infection with other microorganisms) can result in production of factors that reactivate HIV. These secondary infections may be important cofactors in AIDS progression.

3) HIV can carry out infection by *cell-to-cell spread*. That is, if an HIV-infected cell comes into contact with an uninfected cell, the virus may pass to the uninfected cell directly. Neutralizing antibodies are unable to prevent this process, since they can only attack virus when it is outside cells.

These properties of HIV also pose another problem. Vaccines are our front line of defense against most virus infections, as described earlier in this chapter. However, the ability of HIV to evade the immune system means that it will be much more difficult to design an effective anti-HIV vaccine.

AZIDOTHYMIDINE(AZT), AN EFFECTIVE THERAPEUTIC AGENT IN AIDS

One effective drug has been developed against HIV infection and AIDS so far, azidothymidine (or zidorudincor AZT or Retrovir). The effectiveness and use of AZT will be described more in Chapters 5 and 6. However, let's consider its mode of action here.

Azidothymidine is very similar in chemical structure to thymidine, one of the building blocks of DNA. However, when AZT is incorporated in place of thymidine during the DNA assembly process, it aborts further DNA assembly because of its

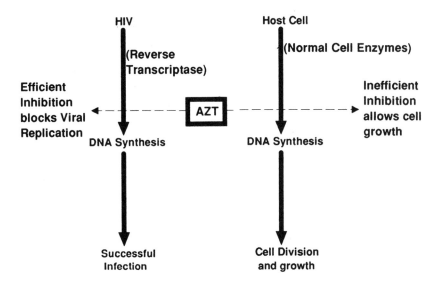

FIGURE 4-11. The action of AZT.

structure. This inactivates any growing DNA molecule that has incorporated AZT. During HIV infection, if AZT is present, HIV reverse transcriptase will readily incorporate it into the viral DNA. This will inactivate the viral DNA. It is important that the enzymes responsible for making the chromosomal DNA of the cell (cellular DNA polymerases) do *not* efficiently incorporate AZT into DNA. As a result, the cell can continue to grow and make its genetic material, but HIV cannot replicated efficiently. Thus, AZT is a *selective poison* for HIV. It exploits an "Achilles heel" of the virus — reverse transcriptase. This enzyme plays no role in the uninfected cell, but it is vital to the virus. An agent that affects this enzyme will have no effect on the uninfected cell, but will inhibit virus infection. This is shown in Figure 4-11.

LIMITATIONS OF AZT. While AZT is an effective drug in AIDS treatment, it has some limitations:

1) *Toxic side effects.* Normal cellular DNA polymerases do not efficiently incorporate AZT into DNA in comparison to HIV reverse transcriptase — the basis for the drug's selectivity. However, cellular DNA polymerases do incorporate some AZT into cell DNA at low levels. During prolonged treatment, this can lead to death of normal cells. Anemia is a common side effect in individuals taking AZT, and results from the killing of blood cells by the drug.

2) *Inability to halt progression to AIDS.* While AZT treatment improves the clinical condition of individuals with Frank AIDS, and also slows progression of asymptomatic people to AIDS, it is not a cure (see Chapter 5). While the exact reason for the inability of AZT to halt progression to AIDS is not understood, one possibility is that the virus may mutate in the individual. Indeed, AZT-resistant HIV has been detected in individuals who have been taking AZT.

Despite its limitations, the effectiveness of AZT in treating AIDS patients has a very important implication. Even in individuals who are already infected, *prevention of continued HIV infection improves the clinical status.* Thus, other drugs that selectively inhibit HIV reverse transcriptase are likely to be useful therapeutic agents, particularly if they can overcome some of the limitations of AZT. Moreover, the other HIV proteins are all potentially "Achilles heels" for the virus as well. Agents that interfere with the action of any of these proteins may also be useful therapeutic agents. AIDS researchers are devoting a great deal of effort to developing new anti-HIV drugs.

WHERE DID HIV COME FROM?

Molecular biologists have examined the genetic structure of HIV (actually HIV-1 and -2) in great detail, and compared it to the structure of other retroviruses of the lentivirus sub-class. From these studies it is clear that HIV shares a common origin with other lentiviruses, and it evolved from a common ancestral retrovirus over millions of years. Epidemiology studies tell us that the HIV that exists today probably evolved to its current form in central Africa hundreds or thousands of years ago. Fifteen to twenty years ago it spread into high density populations in the Western world and Africa, leading to the AIDS epidemic. Recent changes in human social behavior, such as the sexual revolution, may have also contributed to the spread of AIDS.

Numerous apocryphal stories as to the origin of HIV have circulated since the beginning of the AIDS epidemic. These include: HIV was the result of germ warfare research by the CIA; HIV was a laboratory accident involving recombinant DNA; HIV resulted from a plot between Israel and South Africa; HIV resulted from sexual relations between humans and sheep; HIV resulted from sexual relations between humans and monkeys. *None of these is true.*

5

CLINICAL MANIFESTATIONS OF AIDS

Exposure, Infection and Disease
Exposure versus Infection
Infection versus Disease
- Initial Infection and the Asymptomatic Period
  1) Mononucleosis-like Illness
  2) Brain Infection (Encephalopathy)
- Initial Disease Symptoms
  1) Wasting Syndrome
  2) Lymphadenopathy Syndrome
  3) Neurological Disease

Damage to the Immune System and Frank AIDS
- Early Immune Failure
  Candida

Shingles
Hairy Leukoplakia
- Frank AIDS
- Fungal Infections
  PCP
  Systemic Mycosis
- Protozoal Infections
  Cryptosporidium Gastro-enteritis
  Toxoplasmosis
- Bacterial Infections
- Viral Infections
- Cancers

AZT Treatment in AIDS

[77]

I N THE PREVIOUS two chapters we learned about AIDS at the cellular and sub-cellular level.   In particular, cells of the immune system were discussed, and the effects of HIV infection on those cells were presented. With that background we can now consider the effects of HIV in terms of a whole person — the actual symptoms that infected individuals experience. A brief overview of AIDS at the organismal level was included in Chapter 4, and in this chapter a detailed description of the clinical manifestations of AIDS will be presented. While the physical manifestations of the disease are of great importance to AIDS patients and their health-care providers, it is important to remember the human side of the disease as well. Currently AIDS is generally a fatal disease. For people to learn that they are infected with HIV evokes tremendous emotional stress. Counselors trained to help a patient deal with this psychologically difficult situation are important.   In this chapter we will simply present the biological or clinical aspects of AIDS. The psychological consequences of being infected with HIV, or learning that one is HIV-infected, are at least as important but will be considered elsewhere.

EXPOSURE, INFECTION AND DISEASE

In terms of AIDS and HIV at the organismal level, it is important to consider interaction of the virus with a susceptible individual. Three important concepts in the interaction are *exposure, infection* and *disease.*

> **Exposure vs. infection.** When an HIV-infected individual encounters an uninfected person, this does not always result in transmission of HIV to the uninfected person. Indeed, even if exposure occurs by one of the three routes known to transmit the virus (blood, birth, sex), only a fraction of the exposed people will be infected. The relative risk factors affecting the efficiency of HIV transmission will be discussed in Chapters 6 and 7. As we shall see, different kinds of exposure between infected and uninfected individuals have different probabilities of leading to infection.

As introduced in Chapter 4, most individuals who are exposed to HIV and become infected, do not show signs of illness right away. Thus, it is generally not possible to distinguish many infected and uninfected people simply on the basis of their physical well-being. The HIV antibody test is invaluable in identifying individuals infected with HIV (see Chapter 4). Generally, an infected person will begin to produce antibodies against HIV (*seroconvert*) two to three months after infection, although the time for seroconversion is variable and can last as long as six months to a year or more. In practical terms, someone who was exposed to HIV is generally considered to be uninfected if he or she is seronegative for HIV antibodies six months after the last exposure to HIV, and remains seronegative for another six months — during which time no other potential exposures occurred.

Infection vs. disease. Even among individuals who become infected with a virus, not necessarily everybody will develop physical symptoms. For many viruses, most of the infected individuals actually never develop physical signs of illness. Unfortunately, most people infected with HIV ultimately develop some disease symptoms (see Chapter 6).

The disease symptoms that result from virus infection are caused by destruction or damage of cells and tissues in the infected person. In some cases the damage may result from direct killing of cells by the infecting virus. In other cases the physical symptoms may result from indirect effects of the virus. In the case of AIDS, most of the physical symptoms are the indirect results of damage to the immune system by HIV (see Chapters 3 and 4).

Many virus infections can cause a variety of physical symptoms. Other factors can influence the exact nature of the symptoms in a particular individual, including age, sex, genetic makeup, nutrition, environmental factors, and encounters with other infectious agents. As we shall see, this is particularly true for AIDS, where the symptoms result from indirect immunological damage.

Initial Infection

) Transient early (acute) symptoms

Asymptomatic

Initial Symptoms

1. Lymphadenopathy

2. Wasting syndrome / Fever / Night sweats

3. Neurological disease

Early immune failure

1. Shingles (VZV)

2. Thrush (Candida)

3. Hairy Leukoplakia (EBV)

Frank AIDS (Opportunistic infection)

1. Pneumonia (Pneumocystis)

2. Kaposi's sarcoma

3. Other protozoan infections

4. Systemic Fungal infection

5. Bacterial infection (TB like)

6. Viral infection (CMV)

7. Other cancer (lymphoma)

FIGURE 5-1. The progression of symptoms in AIDS.
(The above symptoms may be additive.)

A schematic diagram of the different clinical stages of HIV infection is shown in Figure 5-1. In time sequence, the stages can be grouped into three categories:

1) *Initial infection and the asymptomatic period;*
2) *Initial symptoms;*
3) *Immunological damage* (early signs through Frank AIDS).

INITIAL INFECTION AND THE ASYMPTOMATIC PERIOD. Many people who become infected with HIV never experience any symptoms at the time of initial infection. On the other hand, some HIV-infected people do develop some relatively mild disease symptoms right after infection (prior to seroconversion). These are referred to as *acute* symptoms, and they generally last only a few days and then disappear. Two types of acute symptoms can occur:

1) *Mononucleosis-like illness.* The most common early illness seen with HIV infection resembles another viral disease known as mononucleosis. This illness is not characteristic of a particular virus, in that many other viral infections can cause these symptoms as well. The most prominent symptoms are swollen lymph glands. In the case of HIV infection, this includes lymph glands throughout the body — called generalized *lymphadenopathy.* In addition, there may also be a sore throat, fever and a skin rash. Because these symptoms also result from infection by other viruses, it is not possible to diagnose an HIV infection solely based on the appearance of these symptoms.

2) *Brain infection (encephalopathy).* HIV infection of the brain can occur at this early time and lead to brain swelling or inflammation, particularly of the brain lining or meninges. In medical terms this is called encephalopathy, derived from the Latin for brain inflammation. Macrophage cells in the brain appear to be prominent sites for virus replication during this time. The brain inflammation may result from the influx of immune sys-

tem cells to fight the infection, or the release from infected cells of highly active molecules that can affect other brain cells. An inflamed organ is generally tender and painful. This leads to symptoms of headache and fever. Brain function can be impaired to various degrees. Often the person will have difficulty in concentrating, remembering, or solving problems. There may also be some personality changes during the acute phases.

During the acute phase of infection, significant levels of circulating HIV are generally produced. Following the acute phase the infected person will usually feel well but become seropositive for HIV. This is referred to as the period of *asymptomatic infection*. Generally, circulating levels of infectious HIV are low during the asymptomatic period. Some infected people will not have detectable infectious HIV in their blood and are *latently* infected (see Chapter 4). In these people the HIV genetic information is integrated into the chromosomes of macrophages or lymphocytes but is silent. At some later time, however, the HIV genetic information may become activated and begin to produce virus. Most infected people, however, produce low levels of HIV in their blood and are *persistently* or *chronically* infected. As mentioned above, the asymptomatic period may last longer than eight years or as short as several months. We do not yet understand why there is such variability.

During the asymptomatic period some type of balance apparently exists between HIV infection and the immune system in the infected person. Ultimately, for most individuals changes in the virus or the immune system allow the HIV infection to escape from control and lead to disease.

INITIAL DISEASE SYMPTOMS. The initial disease that follows the asymptomatic period falls into three major classes. An infected person may have symptoms from more than one of these classes. The three classes of symptoms are:

1) **Wasting Syndrome.** The *two* symptoms seen with this syndrome are a sudden and otherwise unexplained *loss*

in body weight (more than ten percent of total body weight) and *fevers* usually at night, which cause *night sweats*. The weight loss is usually progressive leading to the wasting away of the infected person, and may be accompanied by diarrhea. This wasting syndrome is very reminiscent of the progressive loss of body weight by cancer patients. The fevers can involve dangerously high temperatures (106-107 degrees Fahrenheit) that can result in brain damage. Normally the body controls high internal temperatures by sweating. The night sweats result from attempts by the bodies of infected individuals to lower their temperatures.

2) **Lymphadenopathy syndrome.** As described above, lymphadenopathy means swelling of the lymph glands. Lymphadenopathy sometimes is also an acute symptom of HIV infection, but in lymphadenopathy syndrome (LAS), the lymph gland enlargement is persistent. This condition is also called *persistent generalized lymphadenopathy* or *PGL*. In LAS the lymph glands in the head and neck, the arm pits, and the groin are usually swollen, although they generally are not painful. Some infected people will experience both LAS and the wasting syndrome described above. In the past, lymphadenopathy was one of a group of symptoms that was associated with AIDS-related complex (ARC, see Chapter 4), a condition considered less serious than AIDS. However, the term ARC is used less frequently nowadays, and lymphadenopathy actually can occur at various different stages of the disease.

3) **Neurological disease.** The HIV infection can spread to the brain and either damage the brain directly, or lead to damage by other infectious agents. In addition, other parts of the nervous system can be damaged and cause different neurological symptoms. About one third of all AIDS patients will have some of the following neurological symptoms:

Dementias. When the brain itself is damaged mental functions are impaired. With HIV infection this is usually a progressive situation. Initially this may appear as simple forgetfulness about where things are. As the disease progresses the loss of mental function can become more serious: the infected person may have difficulty reasoning and performing other mental tasks. Depression, social withdrawal, and personality changes are also common. Eventually, as the disease progresses infected people may become demented and unable to care for themselves. For some AIDS patients this progression leads to the patient entering a coma followed by death, if other infections or cancers do not kill the patient first. Death from dementia usually occurs several months following the onset of dementia.

Spinal cord damage (myelopathy). Because the spinal chord transmits nerve impulses to the muscles of the body, damage to the spinal chord can result in weakness or paralysis of voluntary muscles. As a result, HIV infection can lead to spinal chord swelling (*myelopathy*) and paralysis or weakness of the limbs.

Peripheral nerve damage (neuropathy). Some people infected with HIV will experience swelling (neuropathy) of the peripheral nerves. These nerves are involved in sensing pain. When they are damaged they can cause burning or stinging sensations, usually in the hands or feet. In addition, the occurrence of numbness, especially in the feet, is frequent.

These initial symptoms of HIV infection are not mutually exclusive. Individual patients may experience a mixture of any of these illnesses.

DAMAGE TO THE IMMUNE SYSTEM AND FRANK AIDS

As described in Chapter 4, the major problem in HIV infection is damage to the immune system. Two major consequences result from immunological damage: the occurrence of *opportunistic infections* caused by infectious agents that are normally held in check by healthy immune systems, and the development of *cancers* that result from failure of immunological surveillance (see Chapter 3). In HIV-infected individuals, both opportunistic infections and cancers may develop (sometimes at the same time), but opportunistic infections are generally the more common causes of death.

As indicated in Chapter 4, the breakdown of the immune system in HIV-infected individuals is a continuous and gradual process. It generally begins with the occurrence of relatively minor opportunistic infections, and usually progresses to severe and life-threatening disease, Frank AIDS. After the isolation of HIV, an early medical definition for diagnosing AIDS was: evidence of HIV infection (seropositivity) in conjunction with two or more serious opportunistic infections or cancers. This was initially useful for epidemiologists and clinicians in staging and classifying the disease. However, we now know that AIDS represents the final and most severe symptoms of HIV infection, and it is not really distinct from other manifestations of the disease. In adults Frank AIDS almost never occurs before two years of infection.

EARLY IMMUNE FAILURE. Previously, the term ARC was sometimes used to describe the relatively minor infections or the lesser manifestations of immune system failure. These are some of the more common opportunistic infections that occur during this time:

> *Candida. Candida* is a species of fungus, similar to bakers yeast, which can be found on the skin and mucosal surfaces (mouth, vagina) of most people. Normally *Candida* growth is held in check by an ecological balance with other microorganisms, and by the immune system. With AIDS patients, Candida will often infect the mouth causing a condition known as Candidiasis or Thrush. With Thrush, the *Candida*

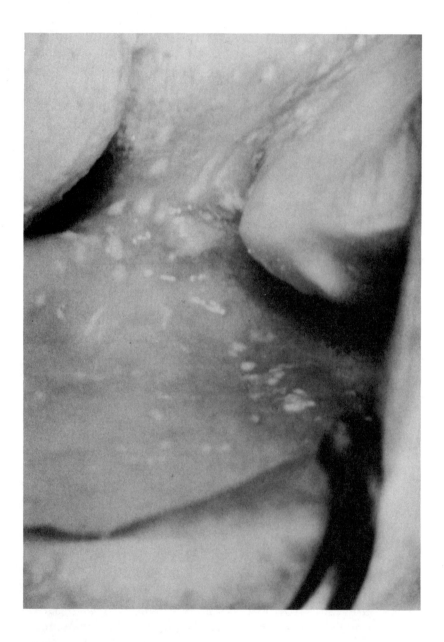

FIGURE 5-2. Oral Candidiasis. The photograph shows the inside of the mouth, with the gums, cheek and tongue (on the right). The white spots are areas of *Candida* (yeast) infection.

will form white plaques in the mouth which feel "furry" to the patient (Figure 5-2). Anti-fungal drugs, such as mycostatin, are used to control these infections, although they are difficult to eliminate completely. HIV-infected people who develop Candidiasis have a high probability of progressing to Frank AIDS. Often the infection can spread down the esophagus and cause a very painful burning sensation when the patient eats. This condition is known as *esophagitis*; patients with esophagitis are generally considered to have Frank AIDS. Approximately 50% of AIDS patients will experience, at some time, a *Candida* infection.

Shingles (varicella). *Shingles* or *varicella* is a painful rash condition, which often occurs on the torso (Figure 5-3). It is caused by the reactivation of a latent virus, called *Varicella zoster*. This is the virus that causes chickenpox during childhood and is a member of the Herpes virus family. After the initial childhood infection, the virus can then remain dormant in the nerve trunks for many years and become reactivated when the immune system is compromised or stressed. With AIDS patients, the severity of shingles appears to be greater than that seen in non-AIDS patients, presumably due to their failing immune systems. The anti-viral drug, acyclovir, is sometimes used to help control shingles.

Hairy leukoplakia. This is an abnormal condition of the mouth in which white plaques appear on the surfaces of the tongue. These plaques are not due to the overgrowth of a fungus or bacteria, however. They are due to the abnormal growth of the papillae cells of the tongue; these plaques cannot be scraped off. These overgrown cells resemble cancer cells and appear to result from infection with another virus called *Epstein-Barr virus*. Epstein-Barr virus is also a member of the Herpes virus family and is the virus that causes infectious mononucleosis in young adults. Hairy leukoplakia condition is a condition unique to AIDS patients.

FRANK AIDS. As discussed elsewhere in this book (Chapters 4 and 6), most HIV-infected individuals will develop some of the

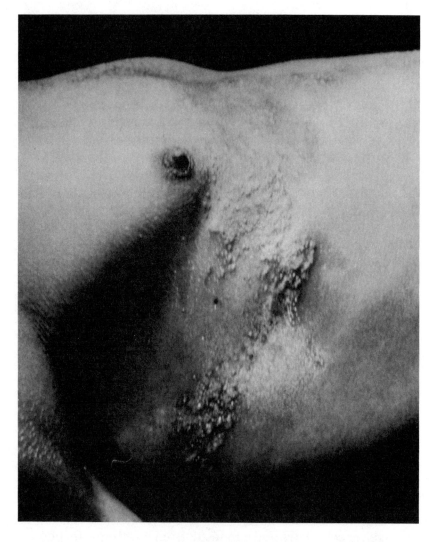

FIGURE 5-3. Shingles. Reactivation of the latent *varicella Zoster* (chickenpox virus) infection is shown in a band across the torso.

symptoms associated with AIDS within eight or more years after initial infection. The rate at which infected individuals develop symptoms may vary somewhat among different risk groups. For instance, hemophiliacs who were infected by transfusions or blood products may develop AIDS at a lower rate than gay men. This may be influenced by the number and nature of other microorganisms (potentially opportunistic infections) that these people encounter. The following infections and cancers seen in AIDS patients are indications that the immune system has undergone a catastrophic failure and can no longer prevent life-threatening infections or cancers:

FUNGAL INFECTIONS:

Pneumocystis **pneumonia (PCP).** This illness, which results from inflammation of the lungs, is by far the most common of the serious secondary infections seen with AIDS. About half of all AIDS patients will eventually develop pneumocystis pneumonia, and it is the leading cause of death in AIDS patients. Inflamed areas of the lungs makes them appear as white spots in lung X-rays (Figure 5-4). The inflammation is caused by infection with fungus called *Pneumocystis carinii.* (Until recently this microorganism was often classified as a protozoan, but it is now considered a fungus, based on molecular biological studies.) This microorganism gets its name from the person who discovered it, Carini, and from the fact that it can grow into cysts in the lungs of rats (pneumo-cystis). *Pneumocystis carinii* is relatively common and small numbers of the fungus can be found in the lungs of healthy people as well as in many animals. It will cause disease in these animals if their immune systems are suppressed. In AIDS patients the infection is often insidious and the patient may be unaware of the seriousness of his illness. A dry cough is common, and a progressive shortness of breath indicates poor lung function. The shortness of breath is due to the inability of the inflamed lungs to take up adequate amounts of oxygen, which can lead to tissue damage throughout the body. *Pneumocystis carinii* particles are detected by staining the fluid washed out of the lungs with a special dye. PCP pneumonia can be treated with various antibiotics called sulfa drugs. The anti-parasitic agents

(a)

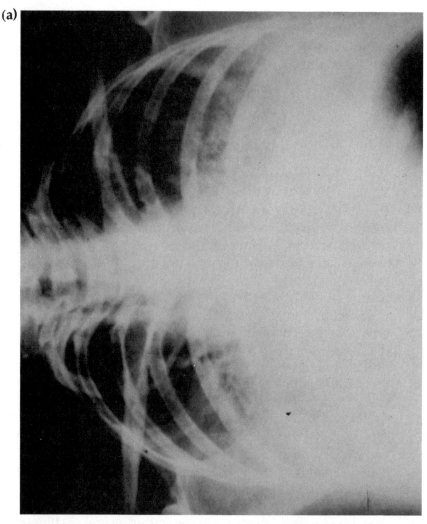

FIGURE 5-4. *Pneumocystis carinii* **pneumonia.** (a) A chest X-ray of an individual with PCP pneumonia is shown. The ribs are apparent in the top of the X-ray, but they are not clear in the bottom. This is because the lungs inside the rib cage are filled with fluid, and they make that area of the X-ray appear lighter. In a normal individual the ribs would be evident against a clear background at the bottom of the picture as well. (*Courtesy of the Center for Disease Control*); (b) Lung tissue from an individual with PCP pneumonia is shown under the light microscope after having been stained. The dark round particles are *pneumocystis* microorganisms within the lung tissue (gray areas).

(b)

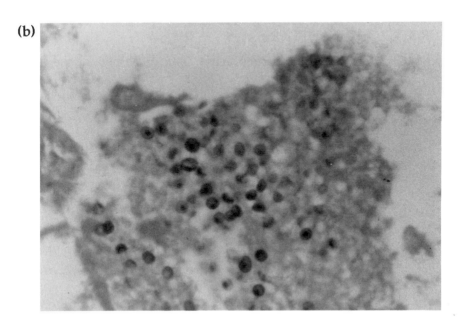

trimethoprim-sulfamethoxazole (TMP-SMX) are usually given together to control the infection. Another drug called pentamidine is also used, especially when TMP-SMX becomes toxic to the patient. Although these antibiotic treatments are often successful, the lung infection can recur. Some drugs (Fancidar) may be given preventively, to prevent recurrences. New drugs, such as trimethexate (an anti-cancer drug), may also be effective against PCP pneumonia.

Systemic mycosis. There are three types of common soil fungi that can cause generalized infections in AIDS patients. These fungi can exist in either a mold- like or yeast-like form, and are called dimorphic. The three types are *histoplasmosis*, *coccidiomycosis*, and *cryptococcus*. These fungi can cause lung infections in healthy people, but generalized or systemic infections are very rare. In AIDS patients, these fungi can cause devastating systemic infections that are massive and very wide spread. The brain, skin, bone, liver, and lymphatic tissue may all be highly infected. This will typically lead to death of the patient. Anti-fungal drugs, such as miconazole, are used to control these infections.

PROTOZOAL INFECTIONS:

Cryptosporidium **gastroenteritis.** This disease is caused by a protozoan called *Cryptosporidium*. This protozoan will infect the linings of the intestinal tract and cause diarrhea (gastroenteritis). In healthy people diarrhea from a *Cryptosporidium* infection is normally mild, lasting only a few days. However, in AIDS patients the diarrhea is prolonged and severe. The AIDS patient may have from 20 to 50 watery stools per day, accompanied by abdominal cramps and profound weight loss. As a result, there is a serious loss of fluid and electrolytes (salts in the blood). For treatment, patients are given fluids and electrolytes intravenously, and their diarrhea can be controlled somewhat with drugs that slow down intestinal action. However, there is currently no standard antibiotic recognized for use against *Cryptosporidium*. Spiramycin, which is currently an experimental drug, may help to control this persistent infection, but it does not eradicate it. Only about 5% of AIDS patients develop this disease. *Cryptosporidium* also infects cattle and other animals, especially their young; these animals may be the source of human infection.

Toxoplasmosis. This disease is caused by species of protozoa called *Toxoplasma gondii*, which normally causes an asymptomatic infection in healthy adults. This protozoan also infects a very wide variety of animals; domestic cats are one source of human infection. Unlike *Cryptosporidium*, *Toxoplasma* is an intracellular parasite and can invade numerous organs of infected individuals. In AIDS patients the brain is often infected, which may result in symptoms similar to that seen with brain tumors: convulsions, disorientation and dementia (Figure 5-5). A CT (computed tomography) scan is used to diagnose toxoplasmosis. For treatment, various antibiotics, such as pyrimethamine and sulfadiazine, are effective, but they must be administered indefinitely to prevent a relapse. Unfortunately, some patients develop a toxic reactions to these drugs.

BACTERIAL INFECTIONS. Interestingly, infections by commonly occurring bacteria (such as those that are in the lower intestines) do not generally occur in adult AIDS patients, perhaps due to the fact that components of the immune system responsible for controlling the common bacteria are less affected by HIV infection. However, children born infected with AIDS often do develop lung infections with common bacteria. In addition, adult AIDS patients may experience infections of tuberculosis-like bacteria.

> *Mycobacterium.* This is a genus of bacteria that has characteristic cell walls with unusual staining properties in the laboratory. The bacterium that causes tuberculosis is a member of this genus. Although AIDS patients may develop tuberculosis, they are more commonly infected with an atypical form of tuberculosis bacterium called *Mycobacterium avium-intracellularae.* This bacterium does not normally cause disease in healthy people, but in AIDS patients it may cause a tuberculosis-like disease in the lungs. The infection can also involve numerous other tissues such as bone marrow, and bacteria may be present in the blood at very high levels (Figure 5-6). Patients with this opportunistic infection will have fevers and low numbers of white blood cells. These infections are often resistant to drugs, and are often treated with the simultaneous administration of up to six different antibiotics. Isoniazid and rifampin are usually among the drugs used. This type of infection is more common in AIDS patients who were IV drug users.

VIRAL INFECTIONS:

> **Cytomegalovirus.** This is a member of the Herpes virus family, as are varicella zoster and Epstein-Barr viruses described previously. Cytomegalovirus (CMV) is a common virus and many people are infected early in childhood. Children tend to get an asymptomatic infection, while infected young adults may develop a mononucleosis-like ill-

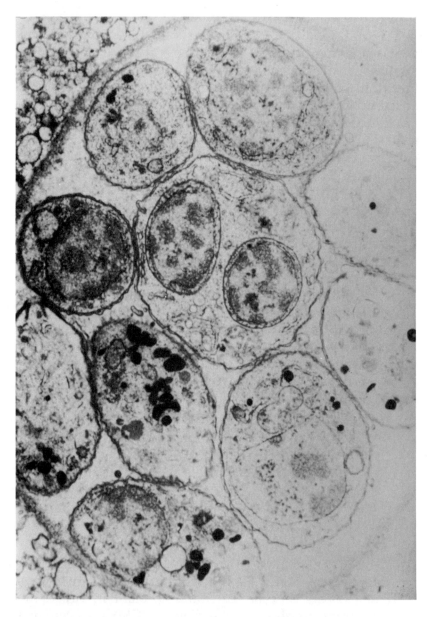

FIGURE 5-5. *Toxoplasmosis.* An electron microscope picture of a *toxoplasma* cyst is shown. A cyst is a walled-off area of microorganisms within a tissue. Each of the round areas in the photograph is a cross-section of a *toxoplasma* microorganism. (*Courtesy of the Center for Disease Control*)

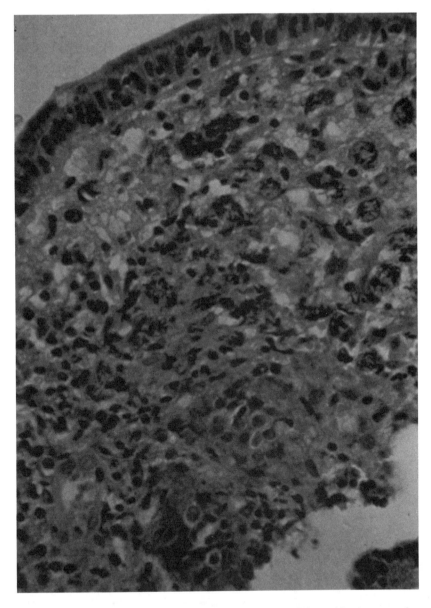

FIGURE 5-6. *Mycobacterium.* A section of the small bowel is shown under the light microscope. The dark particles in the center of the photograph represent *Mycobacterium avium-intracellularae* particles within the bowel tissue. *(Courtesy of the Center for Disease Control)*

ness. Infection of a fetus (a congenital infection) is very serious, and can lead to permanent brain damage or death of the fetus. In AIDS patients CMV infection can recur, and tends to infect the retina of eyes, which leads to blindness. The virus also infects the adrenal gland, which leads to hormonal imbalance. Pneumonia, fever, rash, and gastroenteritis due to CMV infection are also seen in AIDS patients. CMV pneumonia in patients who have PCP pneumonia at the same time is usually fatal. For treatment, the anti-viral drug gancyclovir may help control CMV infections.

CANCERS:

Kaposi's sarcoma. These are tumors of the blood vessels (Figure 5-7). In non-AIDS patients Kaposi's sarcoma (KS) is typically only seen in older men of Mediterranean or Jewish ancestry. In homosexual men with AIDS, up to 69% may develop Kaposi's sarcoma. Initially, only a few tumors appear as pink, purple or brown skin lesions usually located on the arms or legs. These tumors will spread and become widely distributed, eventually involving most of the linings of the body. If they spread to the lungs, they are difficult to control. Chemotherapy can now eradicate these tumors with a high success rate. Triaziquone, actinomycin D, bleomycin and ICRF-159 are often used in chemotherapy. AIDS patients with KS often have a high level of opportunistic infections.

Lymphomas. The lymphomas that occur in AIDS patients are cancers derived from the B-cells of the immune system. These are cells that make antibodies, as discussed in Chapter 3. Reactivation or co-infection in the B-lymphocytes with Epstein-Barr virus may be important for development of the lymphomas. As mentioned previously in this chapter, this Epstein-Barr virus causes mononucleosis in young adults, but it can also transform normal B cells into cancer cells. In AIDS patients, an unusual lymphoma that spreads to the brain also occurs.

This list of opportunistic infections and cancers seen in AIDS patients only covers the most commonly observed diseases. Numerous other infections are also seen at lower frequencies. In addition, an individual patient may experience a mixture of these illnesses. It is interesting that there are characteristic cancers and opportunistic infection in AIDS patients. These diseases are only a fraction of potential diseases that could affect an immuno-compromised person. This may be due to the fact that HIV more seriously damages certain parts of the immune system. In addition, other factors such as previously established chronic or latent infections may be important. Once the immune system fails, these pre-existing infections can then proliferate and cause disease symptoms.

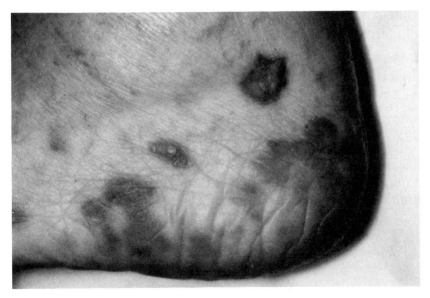

FIGURE 5-7. Kaposi's sarcoma.
Dark (purplish) areas of Kaposi's sarcoma are shown on the heel of the foot.

AZT TREATMENT IN AIDS

In order to restore the health of an AIDS patient it will be necessary to suppress the replication of HIV and to rebuild the damage to the immune system (see Chapter 9). So far this is beyond our technical capacity. Certainly anti-viral drugs will play an important role in the clinical treatment of this disease. Currently only azidothymidine (AZT) is clinically effective in alleviating AIDS (see Chapters 4 and 6). [AIDS patients who are given AZT show increased survival. Without AZT the average life expectancy of an AIDS patient who has an opportunistic infection is about six months. With AZT that life expectancy rises to one and a half years. Treatment with AZT actually results in some recovery of immune function. The number of T_{helper} lymphocytes in AZT-treated AIDS patients increase, they experience fewer opportunistic infections, and may actually gain weight. The patients also feel better.]

For other viral illnesses the infections have never yet been completely eradicated with an anti-viral drug. However, with AIDS it may only be necessary to prevent high levels of virus replication in order to control the disease.

[The cost of AZT is high, about $8,000.00 per year for one person. Current treatment regimens demand that a patient take an AZT pill once every four hours, around the clock, although recent studies suggest that lower doses (half as much) may be effective in some situations.] As mentioned in Chapter 4, AZT treatment has some side-effects, such as nausea, headache, and loss of sleep. The major complication is that about half of treated patients will become anemic and have a low white blood cell count. This in itself can lead to an increase in bacterial infections. If anemia occurs AZT treatment must be discontinued, at least temporarily.

Recent studies indicate that AZT treatment is also effective in asymptomatic HIV-infected individuals. That is, AZT treatment of these people significantly slows the rate at which they progress to clinical AIDS. Moreover, some of the toxic side-effects (anemia) occur less frequently in these individuals. This has led to the general recommendation that individuals who suspect that they may have been exposed to HIV have themselves tested (under conditions that assure counseling and confidentiality). Their immune systems can then be monitored (*e.g.*, T helper lymphocyte counts — see Chapter 4) for signs of damage, and opportunistic infections can be monitored as well. Preventive therapies such as AZT and aerosol pentamidine (to prevent PCP pneumonia) can then be used before the individual becomes seriously ill. Seriously ill patients are much more difficult to treat medically.

6

EPIDEMIOLOGY AND AIDS

I N THE PRECEDING chapter we considered how HIV manifests itself in an infected individual. The next level of complexity will be to consider how HIV moves between individuals, and its effects on populations. For these topics the discipline of epidemiology is very important. The modes of HIV transmission and relative risk factors will be addressed in the following chapter. This chapter gives an overview of epidemiology, with some applications regarding HIV and AIDS.

Epidemiology is the study of the patterns of disease occurrence in populations, and of the factors affecting them. This field is of great importance to the understanding of human diseases, and epidemiological studies can be used to address many questions.

What can epidemiology tell us about diseases? Epidemiological studies can:

1) *Identify new diseases.*
2) *Identify populations at risk for a disease.*
3) *Identify possible causative agent(s) of a disease.*
4) *Identify factors or behaviors that increase risk of a disease.* They can also determine the relative importance of a factor in contributing to a disease.
5) *Rule out factors or behaviors as contributing to a disease.*
6) *Evaluate therapies for a disease.*
7) *Guide the development of effective public health measures and preventative strategies.*

It is important to keep in mind that epidemiological studies involve large groups or *populations* of individuals. This approach gives great power to these studies, since they draw on the total experience and behavior of large numbers of individuals.

The fact that epidemiological studies are based on observation of groups also introduces some limitations and risks in interpretations. One limitation is that these studies cannot predict how any individual person will be affected by a factor even if the population as a whole is affected by that factor. Epidemiological studies also cannot predict the course a disease will take in a particular person. The risks are associated with drawing improper conclusions from epidemiology. For instance, it is important to avoid making an ecological fallacy — explaining behavior of an individual based on observations of an entire group. Another example of improper conclusions is identifying certain characteristics of a group as causing a disease. For example, epidemiological studies have identified male homosexuals as one of the groups at high risk for AIDS. This does not imply that simply being homosexual causes AIDS, as some people have claimed. Instead, certain sexual behaviors by some gay men link them to AIDS, as we shall see later in this chapter and also in Chapter 7.

Despite these limitations and risks, epidemiological studies provide some of the most definitive information about the causes and dynamics of human diseases, short of carrying out experiments on humans.

AN OVERVIEW OF EPIDEMIOLOGY AND AIDS

Epidemiology has played a central role in the fight against AIDS right from the beginning — and this will continue. The initial identification of AIDS as a new syndrome in 1981 was made by epidemiological studies. These studies reported the unusually high occurrence of individuals with rare diseases associated with immunological defects (see Chapter 1). The initial epidemiological studies showed a high frequency of the new disease in sexually active male homosexuals. Furthermore, the pattern of occurrences suggested that AIDS might be caused by an infectious agent that could be transmitted by sexual means. Subsequently, the appearance of AIDS cases among recipients of blood transfusions or blood products (for instance hemophiliacs) as well as intravenous drug abusers suggested that AIDS could be transmitted through contaminated blood. The study of individuals afflicted with AIDS and also of groups of high risk individuals led to the isolation in 1984 of HIV, the virus that causes AIDS. As soon as HIV was isolated, the virus was used to develop the test for HIV antibodies (see Chapter 4). The availability of the HIV antibody test allowed much more accurate epidemiological studies, since evidence of infection could also be detected in healthy asymptomatic individuals. This led to the realization that there are an alarming number of individuals who have been infected with HIV in many parts of the world. Moreover, we are currently only seeing the tip of the HIV iceberg, since it takes several years for the disease to develop. Epidemiological studies of high risk groups have identified the underlying high risk behaviors, such as unprotected sexual intercourse and sharing of IV needles. This in turn has led to development of public health measures and safe-sex guidelines, which are our only weapons in AIDS prevention today. Finally, epidemiological studies (that also could be classified as clinical studies) provided the proof that azidothymidine (AZT) is an effective therapeutic drug for AIDS.

BASIC CONCEPTS IN EPIDEMIOLOGY

There are two basic kinds of epidemiological studies: *descriptive* and *analytical*. The goal of descriptive studies is to describe the occurrence of disease in populations. Analytical studies seek to identify and explain the causes of diseases. Frequently, descriptive epidemiological studies will lead to analytical studies. For instance, descriptive epidemiology may identify a new disease such as AIDS, or suggest hypotheses about the causes of a disease. Interpretation of the descriptive studies will then suggest hypotheses leading to analytical studies that examine the disease in more detail.

Since epidemiology is the study of disease in populations, the proportion of affected individuals in a population is of basic importance. There are two important measures used in epidemiology:

Prevalence. This is the fraction (or proportion) of current living individuals in a population who have a disease or infection at a particular time.

Incidence. This is the proportion of a population who develop *new* cases of a disease or infection during a particular time period.

TABLE 6-1:   HEPATITIS VIRUS INFECTION IN A CITY

	1968	1988
Total population	100,000	150,000
Individuals with hepatitis virus antibodies (seropositives)	500	1,000
Prevalence of seropositive individuals	0.5%	0.67%
	(500/100,000)	(1000/150,000)

Footnote: Note that this is an example for discussion only. There are actually three different viruses which can cause hepatitis.

As an example, let's look at the numbers in Table 6-1. These numbers show individuals with evidence of previous infection with hepatitis virus (antibodies for the virus) in a city for the years 1968 and 1988. During this time the size of the city has also increased from 100,000 to 150,000. The *prevalence* of hepatitis virus infection was .5% in 1968 and it increased to .67% in 1988. The *incidence* of infection during this period was .17% (.67% minus .5%); put another way, this means that per 100,000 people, there were 170 new cases of infection during the twenty year period. The *yearly* incidence rate would be .17% divided by 20 (.0085% or 8.5 new cases per 100,000 people per year). Epidemiologists use these prevalence and incidence data to calculate other expressions of their results, such as risk values.

DESCRIPTIVE STUDIES

Descriptive epidemiological studies measure the appearance of disease by categories of *person, place,* and *time.* An example of disease appearance by person is the observation that lung cancer predominantly appears in individuals who smoke cigarettes (*person* = smokers). Disease appearance by place would be studies showing the low incidence of tooth decay in areas where there is a high level of naturally occurring fluorides in the water supply (*place* = high fluoride areas). Disease appearance by time would be an outbreak of food poisoning resulting from contaminated food at a picnic (*time* = days after the picnic).

An important concept in descriptive epidemiology is *clustering.* Clustering is the unusually high incidence *or* prevalence of a disease in a subpopulation. Clustering can occur by person, place or time, or a combination of them. The first documented outbreak of Legionnaire's disease is a good example of clustering. Legionnaire's disease is a serious bacterial respiratory infection that can be fatal if untreated. The disease was first identified among several members of the American Legion who attended an American Legion convention at a hotel in Philadelphia in the summer of 1976. Thus, the disease was clustered with respect to place (the hotel in Philadelphia), time (1976), and person (American Legion members). Ultimately, a new microorganism (*Legionella*) was isolated that causes Legionnaire's disease.

TYPES OF DESCRIPTIVE EPIDEMIOLOGICAL STUDIES. Descriptive epidemiological studies are carried out according to several design strategies or a combination of these strategies. Two of the important strategies are *case reports* or *case report series*, and *cross-sectional* or *prevalence studies*.

Case reports/case report series. Case reports are descriptions of an unusual disease occurrence in individual patients. Sometimes the nature of the case may also suggest a relationship between some predisposing factor and the disease, or it may also suggest the appearance of a new disease. These suggestions are strengthened if several similar cases are observed and reported together — this is referred to as a case report series. The original report in 1981 by Gottlieb describing PCP pneumonia in six homosexual men is a classical example of a case report series (see Chapter 1). This report suggested that a new disease (AIDS) might be occurring, and that male homosexuals were at high risk.

Cross-sectional/prevalence studies. In these studies a population is monitored for the occurrence of a disease or a series of diseases, and statistics about each case (nature of the patient, geographical location) are recorded. This information can be used to construct a cross-sectional profile for the disease or diseases within the population. These studies are also sometimes carried out over a long period of time, and the date of disease occurrence is also recorded. Once the cross-sectional profile is obtained, then it can be examined for clustering of disease cases by person, place or time. These clusterings can suggest causes of known diseases and also identify new ones.

Cancer registries are an example of these studies. In these registries information is gathered on all cases of cancer occurring in a region. Information from the cancer registry can then be used by cancer epidemiologists to investigate potential causes of cancer. For instance, these registries have provided strong evidence for a causal relationship between cigarette smoking and lung cancer.

The United States Public Health Service maintains a registry of deaths and diseases that is reported on a weekly basis in a journal called the Morbidity and Mortality Weekly Report. Information from this registry was also important in identifying the AIDS epidemic in 1981 and 1982, since there was a sharp increase in cases of PCP pneumonia and Kaposi's sarcoma at that time. The U.S. Public Health Service now publishes a monthly HIV/AIDS surveillance report, which provides current and past epidemiological information exclusively on HIV infection and AIDS.

Prevalence studies can also be used to identify groups within the population that are at higher risk for a particular disease. Besides suggesting possible causes of the disease, this information can be used for other purposes as well. First, if the disease is rare in the overall population it will be more efficient to study the disease by focusing on the high-risk population — this is important for analytical epidemiology (see below). Second, public health workers may want to focus particular attention on the high-risk population as a first step in working out prevention strategies to combat the disease.

ANALYTICAL STUDIES

Analytical epidemiology studies are generally more focused than descriptive studies. They investigate the causes of a particular disease, and they often involve assigning a numerical value to (quantifying) a potential risk factor. In fact, the distinction between descriptive and analytical studies is not absolute. Most epidemiological studies fall somewhere between a completely descriptive study and a purely analytical one. For instance, cancer registries can be used for analytical epidemiology studies in which the relationship between a particular factor and a disease (for instance, smoking and lung cancer) is examined in detail, and the relative risk is determined.

TYPES OF ANALYTICAL EPIDEMIOLOGICAL STUDIES. There are two main approaches to analytical epidemiology, *experimental* or *interventional studies* and *observational studies.*

Experimental/interventional studies. In these studies a condition of an experimental sub-population is changed, and the effect on development of a disease is observed. The results are compared with the main population or an untreated sub-population. This approach has been very useful in testing potential therapies for diseases. For instance, the Salk polio vaccine was tested in a nationwide trial of second and third grade school children in 1953-1954. The success of the trial led to the acceptance of the vaccine and elimination of polio as a major health threat. A more recent example is a test of a vaccine for Hepatitis B virus. This vaccine was tested in a population of sexually active male homosexuals (who are also at high risk for Hepatitis B infection) and shown to be very effective. Clinical drug trials can also be considered interventional epidemiology.

While interventional studies are very useful in testing therapies, it is often difficult to use them to directly test if a factor causes a disease. Treating a group of people with a factor that might cause a disease raises serious ethical questions. This is particularly important if, as in the case for AIDS, there is no effective cure for the disease. One possible solution to this dilemma is to see if the same disease can be induced by the factor in animals. Another approach is that of observational epidemiology.

Observational studies. Observational studies take advantage of the fact that within a population certain individuals will encounter a factor and develop a disease, while others will not. The epidemiologist does not change the conditions of people to study the disease, but rather *subdivides* the population according to possible risk factors or disease and studies them separately. For instance, by subdividing a population into cigarette smokers and non-smokers, the epidemiologist can investigate the effect of cigarette smoking on cancer or heart disease without making anybody smoke. In some cases a properly designed observational study can provide the same information as an interventional study.

There are two main types of observational studies: *case/control* studies, and *cohort* studies.

Case/control studies involve studying a group of individuals with a particular disease (the cases) and comparing them with a group of unaffected individuals (the controls). The controls are often matched for a number of factors not believed to be involved in the disease. If the cases differ from the control by another factor as well, this would suggest that the factor is related to the disease. For instance, if lung cancer patients are compared to individuals without lung cancer, a higher percentage of the cancer patients are cigarette smokers than in the control population.

Case/control studies are particularly useful if the disease being studied only occurs rarely. For instance, if a disease only occurs once per million people in the United States, it would be impractical to survey everybody in the population to study those few cases that occur. On the other hand, there would be about 200 cases of the disease nationally, which could be readily studied by the case/control approach. For the same reason, case/control studies are important at the beginning of infectious disease epidemics when there are still very few cases. The early epidemiology studies in the AIDS epidemic were mainly case/control studies.

Cohort studies focus on a group of individuals who share a particular risk factor for a disease. This group is then examined for the frequency or rate of disease appearance, in comparison to a control population that does not have the risk factor. Such studies can implicate or exonerate a potential risk factor for the disease, and they can also determine the degree to which the risk factor contributes to the disease.

Cohort studies can go forward or backward in time. *Prospective* cohort studies go forward in time, starting with an identified cohort of individuals and documenting development of disease as time progresses. A number of cohort studies for AIDS are presently underway, principally involving gay or bisexual men. For instance, one cohort study involves HIV antibody-positive individuals, and the occurrence of lymphadenopathy syndrome (LAS), ARC and AIDS is being tracked. In another study a group of single men in San Francisco are being followed for infection with HIV, and the factors (sexual practices, IV drug use) associated with infection are being studied.

Cohort studies that go back in time are called *retrospective* studies. In these studies exposure to the risk factor has occurred previously, and the cohort of individuals is later identified for observation. For instance, retrospective cohort studies have been carried out on individuals who worked in asbestos processing plants in the 1940s and 1950s. These individuals subsequently showed a high incidence of lung cancer, implicating asbestos as another potential cause of lung cancer.

CORRELATIONS. In analytical epidemiology results are considered in terms of *statistical associations* or *correlations* between a factor and a disease. For instance, a high frequency of cigarette smoking is found among lung cancer patients, which means there is a statistical association between cigarette smoking and lung cancer. The aim of analytical epidemiology is to deduce *causality* from the statistical association — in our example, that cigarette smoking causes lung cancer. However, there are other possible explanations for statistical associations.

There are three possible reasons for a positive correlation between a factor and a disease:

1) There is no causal relationship. This could result from faulty design of the experiment. For instance, if the control population is not properly matched with the experimental population, a false correlation could be observed.

2) There is an *indirect* relationship. In some situations there may be a third *confounding* variable that influences both the factor being tested and the disease. For instance, there is a positive statistical correlation between alcohol

consumption and lung cancer, but this does not mean that alcohol causes lung cancer. In this case, cigarette smoking is a confounding variable. Cigarette smoking causes lung cancer, *and* cigarette smoking is also statistically associated with alcohol consumption. That is, individuals who are cigarette smokers also tend to drink more alcohol than do non-smokers.

Another example of an indirect relationship is the high statistical correlation between swim suit sales and ice cream sales. This does not mean that ice cream consumption leads to swim suit purchases, or vice versa. In this case summer or high temperature is a confounding variable. More swim suits are bought during the summer when it is warm and beach weather is good, and more people eat ice cream during this time because it is hot.

3) There is a *direct* causal relationship. That is, a change in the factor will lead to a change in occurrence of the disease.

CRITERIA FOR A CAUSAL RELATIONSHIP. In observational studies it is difficult to absolutely prove a causal relationship from a correlation, because the epidemiologist does not change the factor under study. However, there are a combination of criteria that provide tests for causality. These criteria are:

1) *Strength of the association* between the factor and the disease. The strongest correlation would be if everybody with the factor gets the disease, and nobody without the factor gets the disease. A strong correlation makes a causal relationship more likely. The argument is also strengthened if there is a dose-response relationship — that is, if individuals who have received higher exposure to a factor show higher frequencies of disease. However, it is always important to keep in mind that confounding variables could exist (as previously mentioned).

2) *Consistency* of the association. That is, if the same correlation is observed in other studies using different

settings and different populations.

3) The association has the *correct time relationship*. That is, exposure to the agent must occur *before* development of the disease.

4) The association has *biological plausibility*. That is, association of the factor with the disease makes biological sense.

For infectious agents another set of rules has been developed for assessing if a microbe causes a disease, *Koch's postulates*. Koch's postulates are discussed in Chapter 2, and they require both observational and experimental studies. Briefly, a microorganism can be considered the cause of a disease if 1) it is always found in diseased individuals, 2) it can be isolated from the diseased individual and grown pure in culture, 3) the pure microorganism can cause the disease when introduced into susceptible individuals, and 4) the same microorganism can be re-isolated from those individuals.

EPIDEMIOLOGY AND AIDS

Let us now see what epidemiology can tell us about AIDS in more detail. As described in the overview in this chapter, epidemiology has been extremely important in this epidemic. Let's look at some of the epidemiological information, and the conclusions that can be drawn from it.

THE CURRENT PICTURE OF AIDS IN THE UNITED STATES. Figure 6-1 shows the total number of AIDS cases that have been reported in the United States for the years 1981 through 1988. By the beginning of 1990 a total of 131,000 cases had been reported, of which 72,000 have died. Projections for the total number of cases by 1991 are also shown. Current estimates are that between 800,000 and one million people in the U.S. are currently infected with HIV; a sizable fraction of these people are likely to develop AIDS and ultimately die if new therapies are not found. Thus we can see the seriousness of this epidemic, and the strain that it will place on our society.

Figure 6-2 shows the distribution of AIDS cases according to risk groups. Homosexual and bisexual men make up the largest percentage of cases, followed by IV drug users, hemophiliacs and recipients of blood transfusions, sexual partners of HIV-infected individuals, and children of HIV-infected mothers. For a small percentage of cases (about 3%), no risk group has been assigned. However, many of these may be due to the unavailability of information about the patients, or the reluctance of patients to acknowledge membership in a high risk group. Women make up 9% of American AIDS cases; this low percentage is due to the fact that the largest number of cases occur in homosexual and bisexual men. Women make up about half of the AIDS cases for the other risk groups.

The distribution of AIDS cases shown in Figure 6-2 represents the cumulative totals from the beginning of the epidemic. The distribution among different risk groups may change with time. For instance, most of the AIDS cases associated with blood transfusions or blood products resulted from HIV infections before 1985. In 1985, the HIV antibody test became available to protect the nation's blood supply. Now that the risk of infection from blood transfusions has been greatly reduced, the percentage of new AIDS cases resulting from transfusions will decrease in the future. Also, modifications in behavior that decrease high risk behaviors will change these percentages. In San Francisco a concerted educational campaign targeted at the gay male community has markedly reduced the rate of new HIV infections in that high risk group. On the other hand, if HIV infection spreads further within high risk groups or into other populations, then cases among these groups will increase. For instance, HIV infection is currently spreading virtually unchecked among IV drug users in the New York City - New Jersey metropolitan area. In this area more than 70% of individuals who use IV drugs are HIV-infected. Indeed, in this area IV drug users make up a majority of the *new* AIDS cases. At the present time other geographical areas have lower rates of HIV infection in the IV drug user population, but if

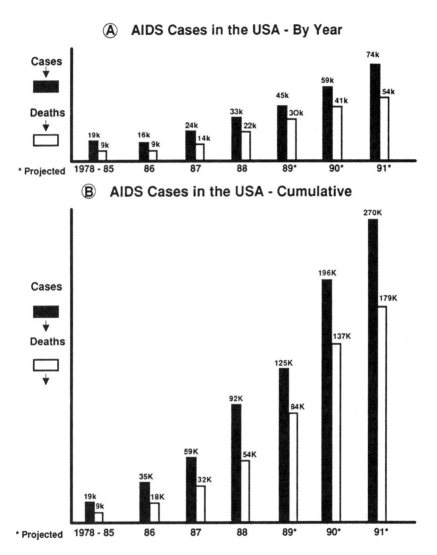

FIGURE 6-1. Appearance of AIDS in the USA.

infection spreads in these areas, then a marked shift in distribution of AIDS cases may occur.

Figure 6-3 shows the distribution of AIDS cases according to ethnicity. There is a disproportional number of AIDS cases among minorities, particularly Blacks and Hispanics. Indeed, while these

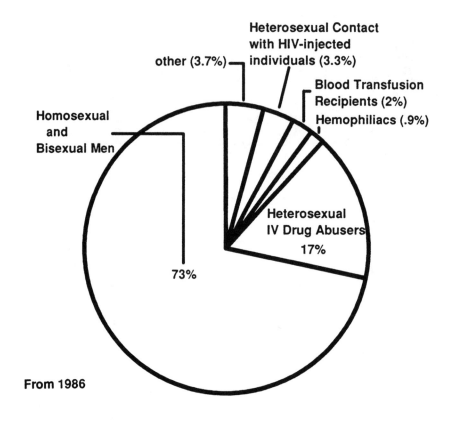

FIGURE 6-2. Distribution of AIDS cases by risk groups.
(Cumulative figures, 1981-January, 1990)

groups make up about 23% of the general population, they make up 43% of AIDS cases — and an even higher percentage of the cases associated with IV drug abuse. Put another way, the frequency of AIDS cases among Blacks and Hispanics is about twice as high as in the general population. This points out the urgency of developing public health and educational measures targeted to these communities in order to control the epidemic.

EPIDEMIOLOGY AND MODES OF HIV TRANSMISSION. Transmission of HIV will be addressed in detail in the next

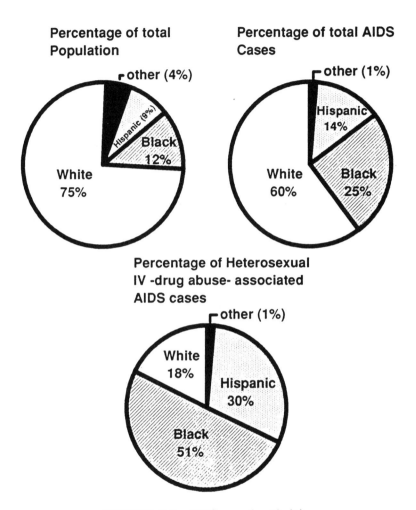

Percentage of total
Population

other (4%)

Hispanic (9%)

Black
12%

White
75%

Percentage of total AIDS
Cases

other (1%)

Hispanic
14%

White
60%

Black
25%

Percentage of Heterosexual
IV -drug abuse- associated
AIDS cases

other (1%)

White
18%

Hispanic
30%

Black
51%

FIGURE 6-3. AIDS cases by ethnicity.
(Cumulative figures, 1981-January, 1990)

chapter. However, some examples of epidemiological studies regarding HIV transmission will be presented here to illustrate how these studies allow us to draw conclusions about the relative risks of different activities for HIV transmission. One study will implicate an activity (anal sex) in HIV transmission, and another study will show that casual contact does not cause HIV transmission. In addition, the possibility of HIV transmission by insects will be considered.

Anal sex — a high risk mode. Let's consider a recent epidemiological study that looked at the relative risks of different sexual activities. This study was part of the San Francisco Men's Health Study (see also Chapter 7), which is an ongoing cohort study of single men in an area of San Francisco. This particular area has been particularly hard-hit by the AIDS epidemic. The study involves 1034 single men who are monitored for HIV antibody status and asked about their sexual practices. Of the homosexual men in this cohort, 48% were seropositive at the beginning. A low percentage (17.6%) of men who had refrained from sex during the previous two years were seropositive, and this could be traced to sexual activity before that time. Table 6-2 shows frequencies of HIV infection when the homosexual men in the study were divided according to whether they practiced anal intercourse. Those who were the receptive partner or who were both receptive and insertive showed significantly higher frequencies of HIV infection than those who did not engage in anal sex. This shows that anal intercourse is a high risk mode of HIV infection.

The results also showed that those who only practiced insertive anal intercourse were at less risk — in fact, this particular study could not statistically distinguish those men from men who did not engage in anal sex at all. However, other studies of heterosexual couples (who engage in vaginal as well as anal intercourse) clearly show that insertive intercourse can result in HIV transmission to the man. Thus, the most likely situation is that anal receptive intercourse is a very high risk sexual activity, while insertive intercourse is somewhat lower, although significant, in risk.

Casual contact—no measurable risk for HIV transmission. *Casual contact* with HIV-infected individuals poses no risk for infection. This was determined early during the epidemic, since people living with AIDS patients did not develop signs of HIV infection or AIDS. Casual contact includes hugging,

EPIDEMIOLOGY AND AIDS 119

TABLE 6-2: HIV INFECTION IN HOMOSEXUAL MEN:
THE RELATIVE RISK OF ANAL SEX

Sexual Practices for the Preceding 2 Years	% HIV Seropositive (Adjusted for Number of Sexual Contacts
No Anal Sex	20.6%
Anal Sex -- Insertive Only	26.7%
Anal Sex -- Receptive Only	44.6%
Anal Sex -- Both Insertive and Receptive	53.3%

Footnote: These data are from the San Fransisco Men's Study, as reported by Winkelstein *et al.* (J. Amer. Med. Assoc. 257:321 [1987]). Individuals who did not practice anal sex for the previous two years included those who practiced oral sex only, and also those who abstained entirely. The strongest correlation for HIV seropositivity in this study was the number of sexual contacts that an individual had. The percentages in the table were adjusted to account for the average number of sexual contacts for the different groups.

touching, dry kissing, sharing of eating or drinking utensils, sharing the work place, telephones, etc.

An example of an epidemiological study establishing that casual contact does not lead to HIV infection is shown in Table 6-3. One hundred and one individuals who shared a household with an AIDS patient for at least three months were tested for the presence of HIV antibodies. Only one person was seropositive, and this individual was a child of two IV drug users. Further tests showed that this child acquired the infection prenatally and not through casual contact. Thus, none of the individuals in this study became HIV-infected through casual contact.

Insect bites — no evidence of spread of HIV. Some people have claimed that insect bites can be a source of infection, because insects such as mosquitoes draw a blood meal from

TABLE 6-3:   HIV INFECTION IN CASUAL HOUSEHOLD CONTACTS OF
AIDS PATIENTS

	Number Tested	Number HIV Seropositive
Children less than 6 Years Old	21	1*
Offspring of an AIDS Patient	15	1*
Offspring of Others	6	0
Children 6 to 18 Years Old	47	0
Adults	33	0
Total tested	101	

Footnote: The subjects in this study had lived in the same household with an AIDS patient for at least three months. Individuals who were in known high risk groups (sexual relations with the AIDS patient, IV drug abuse, homosexual men) were not included. Thus only individuals who had casual contact with the AIDS patient were studied. Among this group, 48% shared drinking glasses with the AIDS patient, 25% shared eating utensils, 9% shared razor blades, 90% shared toilets and 37% shared beds. The AIDS patient was hugged by 79% of the subjects, kissed on the cheek by 83%, and kissed on the lips by 17%. *Further investigation showed that the one seropositive child was the offspring of two IV drug abusers, and probably acquired the infection at birth -- this is a known mechanism of HIV transmission. Thus, none of these casual household contacts of AIDS patients became infected. These data are taken from a report by Friedland et al. (New England J. Med. 314:344 [1986]).

a person that they are biting, and they move from person to person. However, epidemiological evidence argues against insect transmission of HIV. First of all, in well-studied North American or European populations the great majority (about 97%) of AIDS cases can be explained by the well-documented modes of transmission. This includes a recent study in Belle Glade, Florida, where some people proposed an outbreak of AIDS due to insect transmission. Furthermore, in Africa, where the insect populations are high, the age and geographical distributions of HIV infection argue against insect transmission. HIV is rare in children and the elderly, even in households where there are HIV-infected individuals. The old and the young are actually more frequently bitten by mosquitoes and other insects. In terms of geographical distribution, HIV infection is at high frequency in certain cities and urban areas, and there is much lower frequency of infection in surrounding rural areas. This is actually opposite from the pattern that would be expected if insects transmitted HIV since they are more plentiful in rural areas.

LIKELIHOOD OF PROGRESSION TO AIDS. One very important question is the likelihood of an HIV-infected individual eventually developing clinical AIDS. Initial estimates were that perhaps 10% of infected individuals would develop the disease. However, more recent studies indicate that a much higher percentage of infected individuals will develop the disease. Prospective cohort studies have followed HIV seropositive individuals for development of AIDS or ARC. An example of one study is shown in Table 6-4. After about four years of observation, 18% of the seropositive individuals developed AIDS, and an additional 47% developed signs of immunological impairment. Only 35% remained asymptomatic. Other similar studies currently predict that most individuals infected with HIV (more than 70%) will develop AIDS or ARC within eight or more years of infection.

THE EFFECTIVENESS OF AZT. As described in Chapter 3, azidothymidine (AZT) is the only recognized anti-viral agent effective in AIDS. Previous laboratory experiments had shown that the drug could block HIV infection in isolated culture systems, and the drug was tested in a clinical trial that can also be considered an interventional epidemiological study. AIDS patients who had experienced one bout of *pneumocystis* pneumonia were divided into two groups. One group received AZT while the

TABLE 6-4: LONG-TERM RESULTS OF HIV IN INFECTED MEN

	Number of Individuals	% Total
AIDS	10	17.5%
Signs of Immunological Damage		
LAS	16	28.1%
Others (Oral candidiasis, weight loss, etc.)	11	19.3%
Sub-total	27	47.4%
Asymptomatic	20	35.1%

Footnote: Men in this study were followed for an average of 44 months after they showed initial signs of HIV infection (seroconversion). These data are taken from Ward *et al.* ("AIDS", G.P. Worser *et al.* eds., Noyes Publications, Park Ridge, NJ [1987]. pp18-35).

other control group received "placebo" pills that contained no drug. The physical states of all of the subjects were then monitored on a regular basis. As shown in Table 6-5, after the study was in progress for six months the results showed markedly better survival of the group taking AZT than the control group. In fact, the results were so striking that the investigators terminated the trial early and administered AZT to the control patients as well. Withholding the drug would have been unethical at that point. These studies led to approval of AZT for therapy in AIDS. Other studies are now in progress to test different administration routines for AZT and its use in other AIDS-related conditions (see Chapter 5). Other possible anti-viral drugs are being tested as well.

TABLE 6-5: EFFECT OF AZIDOTHYMIDINE TREATMENT ON SURVIVAL OF AIDS AND ARC PATIENTS

Treatment	Number of Subjects	Number of Deaths	% Deaths
None (Placebo pills)	97	19	19.6%
AZT	124	1	0.8%

Footnote: The subjects were in the study an average of 16 to 17 weeks. The study was intended to last 24 weeks (6 months), but it was terminated early, once the dramatic effect of AZT treatment became evident. All subjects were offered AZT at that time. These data are taken from the report of the first large-scale test of AZT (Fishl *et al.*, New England J. Med. 317:185 [1987]).

AIDS IN AFRICA

As mentioned previously, AIDS is also a major health problem in sub-Saharan Africa. The disease is centered in countries of central Africa, including Zaire, Kenya, Uganda, Zambia and Rwanda. In contrast to the distribution of cases in North America and Europe, HIV infection is distributed equally among men and women, and epidemiology reflects the fact that a predominant mode of transmission is heterosexual intercourse. Other modes of transmission may include blood transfusions, injections with reused needles, and procedures that involve scraping of the skin with surgical knives (scarifications). The epidemic probably spread along truck routes through central Africa, and female prostitutes have been important reservoirs for the infection. The AIDS epidemic is mostly concentrated in cities and urban areas, and is much lower in rural areas. As in North America and Europe, the spread of HIV infection in Africa is a recent phenomenon, mostly occurring in the 1980s.

The extent of HIV infection in sub-Saharan Africa is alarmingly high. For example, as many as 90% of female prostitutes in Nairobi, Kenya are HIV-infected today. In 1985-1986 18% of men visiting venereal disease clinics in Nairobi were seropositive for HIV, and the percentage has rapidly climbed since then. As many as 25% of the sexually active populations of some cities in Rwanda may be infected. There may be ten million HIV-infected individuals in Africa, most of whom will probably progress to AIDS and eventually die. This will have devastating social and economic impact on these countries, and may reach the proportions of some of the ancient epidemics described in Chapter 2.

Recently another virus related to HIV has also been discovered in Africa. In fact, the original HIV that is associated with the great majority of AIDS cases is called HIV-1 (see Chapter 4). The new virus is called HIV-2 and is predominantly found in countries along the west African coast, such as Senegal and the Ivory Coast. Molecular biological experiments tell us that HIV-1 and HIV-2 are closely related but distinct viruses that evolved from a common ancestor hundreds or thousands of years ago. HIV-2 also causes AIDS, although there are some indications that it is less able to cause disease than HIV-1. The existence of HIV-2 raises a problem since the standard HIV-1 ELISA tests will not detect HIV-2 antibodies. Thus the standard HIV test will not detect individuals infected with HIV-2. So far in North America only one case of HIV-2 infection has been found. However, it may be important to screen blood supplies and individuals for HIV-2 infection as well, in order to avoid undetected contamination or infections.

7

MODES OF HIV TRANSMISSION AND PERSONAL RISK FACTORS

Biological Bases of HIV Transmission
- Sources of Infectious HIV
- Stability of HIV
- Targets of HIV Infection

Modes of HIV Transmission
- No Association with HIV Transmission: Casual Contact
- Activities associated with HIV Transmission

- Receiving a Transfusion of Blood or Blood products
- Prenatal Transmission
- HIV-infected Syringes
- Sharing Needles
- Accidental Needle Sticks
- Intimate Sexual Contact
- Safer Sexual Practices
- Less Risky Sexual Practices
- Risky
- Dangerous

I N PREVIOUS chapters we have analyzed how the AIDS virus operates at the cellular level as well as at the organism level. Now our focus shifts to the inter-organism level. In this chapter we will look specifically at the question of how HIV is transmitted from person to person. Because there currently is no cure for AIDS once an individual has contracted the disease, preventing the transmission of HIV from person to person is critical. In this chapter, consequently, we shall consider risk factors for HIV transmission and discuss ways for reducing these risk factors.

The evidence for assigning risks to different levels of activities comes from two main sources: theoretical biological considerations and empirical epidemiological data, bolstered by laboratory data. Theoretical analysis considers the biological plausibility of HIV transmission for particular activities based on the presence or absence of substances containing HIV and of receptors for these substances. For example, we know that HIV is not present in someone's exhaled breath; consequently, on the basis of theoretical analysis alone, we would assign little risk to breathing the air in the same room with a person with AIDS.

Theoretical analysis can be used to make predictions about no-, low- or high-risk activities. These ultimately can be tested by empirical epidemiological data, the other main source of evidence for our risk judgments in this chapter. To continue the example above, epidemiological data from the sample of individuals who have lived with people with AIDS provides corroborating evidence that breathing the same air does not spread HIV (see Chapter 6). Because epidemiological data indicates no AIDS incidence among family and friends who have simply lived with AIDS patients and because of the biological implausibility, we can confidently state that breathing the same air is not a risk factor.

Typically, it is activities with a high biological plausibility for HIV transmission that are carefully investigated with epidemiological studies. We saw one example in the last chapter. Anal receptive sexual activity has a high biological plausibility of HIV transmission, and the evidence from epidemiological studies discussed in Chapter 6 provided corroborative evidence that this behavior is in fact strongly associated with HIV infection.

In addition, epidemiological evidence can provide the initial evidence that certain activities are or are not associated with HIV infection risk. At the outset of the AIDS epidemic, for instance, it was epidemiological studies that led to the identification of likely modes of HIV transmission. This in part guided subsequent biological laboratory work, aided in the theoretical understanding of AIDS, and resulted in the isolation of HIV.

We should remember one aspect of epidemiological information at the outset of our discussion of risk and risk factors. Epidemiological studies have identified certain groups of individuals who are overrepresented in the population of those with AIDS: in particular, gay and bisexual men and IV drug users make up a large percentage of those with AIDS. There is nothing about being gay, bisexual or an IV drug user that, by itself, leads to HIV infection and AIDS. Rather, these groups of individuals are, on average, more likely to undertake certain behaviors that have a high biological plausibility of HIV transmission. In addition, because of the greater prevalence of HIV infection among people in these groups, the likelihood of transmission is increased if the necessary and sufficient behaviors for HIV transmission occur.

Consider, for example, two cases: a homosexual man (Jim) who has unprotected anal sex with another homosexual man, and a heterosexual woman (Susan) who has unprotected vaginal sex with a heterosexual man. Assume that neither Jim nor Susan is HIV positive. In each case, Jim and Susan are involved in behaviors that have a high biological plausibility for HIV transmission. The important and unknown factor, then, is the HIV status of their partner. On the sole basis of *average* HIV infection rates, which are higher among gay men as a group than among heterosexual men as a group, Jim is at more risk than Susan. However, without complete data on their partner's HIV status and sexual history, neither Jim nor Susan can be certain of their risk for this particular sexual encounter. The safest approach, as we shall see in the following pages, is to avoid unprotected anal or vaginal intercourse.

Before we consider the risks of particular behaviors, however, we need to understand the biological bases of HIV transmission, including such issues as the primary sources of HIV within an infected person, the stability of the virus in moving between individuals, and the targets for infection in an uninfected individual.

BIOLOGICAL BASES OF HIV TRANSMISSION

In infected people infectious HIV is present only in cells and human body fluids. Despite its devastating effects within the body, the virus is actually quite fragile in the external environment and dies quickly when exposed to room temperature and air conditions. In fact, very special laboratory conditions are needed to grow HIV outside the human body. It is important to remember this fact because it is easy to assume mistakenly that a disease as deadly as AIDS must be caused by an agent that is tremendously strong and sturdy. Peoples' fears of the disease, combined with their lack of knowledge and mistaken impressions about epidemics, can cause them to view HIV in an anthropomorphic way—almost like a living, breathing enemy capable of thought and devastating action. Instead, the reality of HIV outside the body is much different: a fragile virus that loses infectivity quickly.

SOURCES OF INFECTIOUS HIV. In an infected individual HIV is present in certain cells as well as in bodily fluids and secretions, many of which also contain these cells. In terms of cells, macrophages and T-helper lymphocytes are susceptible to infection by HIV, as described in Chapter 4. Macrophages may be the long term reservoirs of HIV in infected individuals since they are not killed by the virus. In terms of distribution in the body, macrophages circulate through the blood stream, and they also are found in all mucosal linings of the body, such as the internal urogenital surface of the vagina and penis, the lining of the anus, lungs and throat.

Among people who test positive for HIV, the virus is not found consistently in all body fluids and products. Furthermore, in body fluids where HIV is regularly found, it occurs in different concentrations at different times. Nonetheless, we can place the body fluids and products into two groups: those where HIV is present regularly enough and in sufficient concentrations to be a threat, and those where it is not. Table 7.1a lists these groups and each is discussed in more detail below.

Researchers have developed methods to test for HIV and estimate the amounts of infectious virus present in various body fluids and secretions (see Chapter 4). HIV can be isolated relatively easily from blood (including vaginal and cervical secretions and menstrual fluid) and semen. It has also been isolated from breast milk. With much greater difficulty the virus has also been isolated from saliva, tears, perspiration, urine and feces. The amounts of HIV in these latter body fluids and products are probably 100 or more times lower than for blood or semen. The current scientific view is that body fluids and products other than blood, semen and breast milk contain so little if any HIV that they are not of major importance in HIV transmission between individuals.

Blood and semen in particular are of greatest concern when we consider HIV transmission. When blood and semen are examined closely, the great majority of HIV is associated with infected cells (mostly macrophages) present in these fluids. In the case of blood, if the cells are removed low levels of HIV are present in the cell-free serum. In the case of semen, if the sperm cells and white blood cells are removed HIV is not present in the cell-free seminal fluid.

The relative HIV infectivity of different body fluids and products can be explained in another way from biological considerations. The fluids and products listed in the two groups in Table 7.1a differ in the amount of live cells they contain. Blood, semen, vaginal and cervical secretions and breast milk contain high numbers of live cells. The other body fluids and products (saliva, tears, perspiration, urine and feces) are completely or nearly completely free of live cells (although they may contain non-human cells such as bacteria). Since live infected cells produce HIV, we would expect fluids with live cells to pose the greatest risks for HIV transmission.

STABILITY OF HIV. For transmission of HIV infection to occur, infectious virus must survive long enough to pass to a susceptible person and infect target cells. The structure of the HIV virus particle (see Chapter 4) is actually a very fragile one, as previously

TABLE 7.1a: INFECTIVITY OF DIFFERENT BODY FLUIDS AND
PRODUCTS

Group 1: High HIV Infectivity

Blood

Semen

Vaginal and Cervical Secretions, including menstrual fluid

Breast Milk

Group 2: Low HIV Infectivity

Saliva

Tears

Perspiration/Sweat

Urine

Feces

TABLE 7.1b: HIV INFECTION IN HOMOSEXUAL MEN:
RELATIVE RISK OF ORAL SEX

Sexual Practices for the Preceding Two Years	Percent HIV Seropositive (Adjusted for Number of Sexual Contacts)
No Sex	22.0 %
Oral Sex Only	24.7%

Note: Data from the San Francisco Men's Study, as reported by Winkelstein et al. (J. Amer. Med. Assoc. 257;321 [1987]). HIV infection in the men who had not had sex for the previous two years could be attributed to anal sex prior to that time.

discussed. In particular, the viral envelope is delicate. As a result the virus quickly becomes inactivated when exposed to drying effects of air or light. It is also quickly inactivated by contact with soap and water.

As mentioned above, much of the infectious HIV is associated with cells (macrophages). In blood or semen cells will maintain infectious HIV as long as they themselves are alive. Thus, intravenous transfusions or sexual intercourse involving HIV-infected individuals efficiently transmits infection, since live cells are passed. On the other hand, if blood or semen is allowed to dry the cells die quite quickly and the HIV infectivity is lost.

These facts about the stability of HIV, combined with the facts about likely sources of HIV infection, explain why casual contact with people with AIDS does not result in the spread of HIV infection (see Chapter 6 and the following pages).

TARGETS FOR HIV INFECTION. At the cellular level HIV infection requires the presence of virus receptors on the cell surface. As described in Chapter 4, the receptor for HIV is the CD4 surface protein, which is only present on T-helper lymphocytes and macrophages. Thus, these are essentially the only kinds of cells that become infected in a susceptible individual. These cells are most abundant in the blood. Consequently, activities that introduce infectious HIV, either as infected cells or free virus, into the blood of an uninfected individual will potentially result in infection. For example, sexual intercourse can result in damage or tears (sometimes microscopic) of the mucosal linings of the male or female genital tracts or of the anus. These tears can allow passage of blood or semen into the circulatory system of the uninfected individual. In addition, as described above, macrophages are also present at the mucosal surfaces of the anus and genital tract, and they potentially can be infected directly without the necessity of virus entry into the blood stream.

There is another potential target for HIV infection: the oral cavity and the throat. Like the genital tract and the anus, the throat has a mucosal lining that contains macrophages. In certain sexual activities, such as oral sex, semen is exchanged orally from one person to another. Consequently, there is the theoretical potential for infection. The epidemiological reality, however, is that oral sex is not a primary mode of transmission of HIV. The explanation for this may be that there is less physical trauma associated with oral sex or that physiological features of the oral cavity reduce the efficiency of transmission. This case demonstrates the need to combine theoretical predictions from biological facts with epidemiological data about actual incidence rates in order to understand fully the risks of actual HIV transmission. It is this topic to which we now turn.

MODES OF HIV TRANSMISSION

We are now ready to analyze the modes of HIV transmission from person to person and the relative risks associated with different modes. In making our assessment of risk, we will rely on both the plausibility of HIV transmission, based on theoretical biological analysis, and the empirical facts associating documented HIV transmission with various modes drawn from epidemiological studies. Together, these two sources of information permit us to categorize activities and behaviors according to the degree of their association with HIV infection.

NO ASSOCIATION WITH HIV TRANSMISSION: CASUAL CONTACT. Because HIV is so fragile outside the body, transmission requires *direct* contact of two substances: fluid containing infectious HIV from an infected person and susceptible cells (usually via the bloodstream) of another person. Because of the absence of this type of direct contact, a large group of interpersonal activities and behaviors, generally referred to as "casual contact," have no measured association with HIV transmission (see Chapter 6) and therefore pose no risk for HIV infection.

What do we mean by "casual contact?" This includes all types of ordinary, every-day, non-sexual contacts between and among people. Shaking hands, hugging, kissing, sharing eating utensils, sharing towels or napkins, using the same telephone and using the same toilet seat are a few examples of casual contact. It is impossible to list all types of casual contact here, but we can analyze or make predictions about others, keeping in mind the need for direct contact with body fluids containing infectious HIV. For example, consider the possibilities of water- or air-borne transmission. Because HIV is quickly inactivated outside the body, it cannot survive in the open air or in water. Consequently, we would predict that there is no risk in sharing the same physical space with a person with AIDS or swimming in the same pool. Epidemiological evidence supports this conclusion: there is no measured risk of transmission.

ACTIVITIES ASSOCIATED WITH HIV TRANSMISSION. HIV transmission needs to occur directly between HIV-tainted fluid from an infected person into the blood stream or onto a mucosal lining of another person. Epidemiological data point to four modes of HIV transmission from person to person. These are listed in Table 7.2 and discussed in the rest of this chapter.

TABLE 7-2: MODES OF HIV TRANSMISSION

---

1. **Receiving a blood transfusion with HIV-infected blood.**

2. **Perinatal transmission between an infected mother and a gestating infant.**

3. **Contact with HIV-infected syringes.**

4. **Intimate sexual contact with an HIV-infected person.**

RECEIVING A TRANSFUSION OF BLOOD OR BLOOD PROD-
UCTS. Since a transfusion involves placing foreign blood directly
into the recipient's blood stream, the necessary conditions for HIV
transmission are present: direct contact of potentially infected
fluid with susceptible cells in the recipient. Prior to 1985, when
screening of the blood supply for HIV by the antibody test was
begun (see Chapter 4), the sufficient condition for contracting
AIDS was present: HIV-infected blood for transfusion. Even then,
the risk was low that the blood or blood product involved in a
transfusion was infected — except for hemophiliacs who required
numerous transfusions. Now, however, this sufficient condition
is very unlikely.

It is estimated that 18 million units of blood components are
transfused per year in the U.S. In 1984, the year before antibody
test screening of the blood supply was begun, it is estimated that
7,200 persons were infected with HIV via infected blood or blood
products. Now the estimate is that, at most, 460 people a year will
receive infected blood or blood products. These cases are due to
the fact that the screening tests are not perfect, or the possibility
that detectable antibodies have not yet developed in a recently
infected donor. Consequently, the risk of receiving HIV-infected
blood or blood products now is 2.55 out of 100,000, compared to
the 1984 risk of 40 out of 100,000. Compared to the risk of dying
for a person who is hospitalized and requires a transfusion but
does not receive it (that is, 40 out of 100, or 40,000 out of 100,000),
the risk of receiving HIV–infected blood during a transfusion is
about 15,500 times less.

There are ways to reduce the risk even further. In addition to
routine screening using the tests discussed in Chapter 4, new
information campaigns have been developed that discourage
blood donation from those who might be infected. New procedures also have been established to permit donors, particularly
those who may feel pressured during a work-associated blood
drive, to indicate confidentially that their blood should not be
used. The American Red Cross blood donation offices give all
blood donors a special card describing a procedure that must be
followed by all potential donors. The card lists nine groups of
people who should not give blood, then describes a confidential

procedure that all donors must follow, involving bar-code labels indicating "transfuse" or "do not transfuse." People in one of the nine groups (*e.g.*, drug users, men who have had sex with men since 1977) are to remove the "Do not transfuse" bar code tag and place it on another card. Those not in one of the listed groups remove the "transfuse" bar code tag and place it on the card. To the casual observer the bar code tags are identical, but not to the optical scanner that later identifies blood to be rejected. As these procedures become routinely accepted by staff and donors, the risk of receiving infected blood or blood products from a transfusion will become even smaller.

PERINATAL TRANSMISSION BETWEEN AN INFECTED MOTHER AND HER GESTATING INFANT. This mode of HIV transmission poses a much greater risk than the previous mode. The two necessary conditions are present: HIV-infected blood in the mother's bloodstream and the potential ability of the virus to move between the mother's and child's bloodstreams. In fact, the mother's and child's bloodstreams are technically separated by the placenta, which prevents exchange of cells but not of nutrients and smaller particles like viruses. HIV can potentially pass through the placenta from the mother into the infant's bloodstream and thus infect the infant. Also, during the third trimester of pregnancy small tears sometimes occur in the placenta that can lead to entry of cells from the mother's bloodstream into the child. In addition, during birth itself the child frequently comes into close contact with the mother's blood due to the bleeding associated with delivery. Current statistics indicate that there is about a 50% chance that a child from an infected mother will be infected. The dilemmas that this fact poses for HIV-infected women who want to be mothers (and for society as a whole) are not easy ones.

CONTACT WITH HIV-INFECTED SYRINGES. There are two ways that HIV-infected needles could lead to transmission: when needles are shared during intravenous (IV) drug use and through accidental needle sticks between HIV-infected individuals and health workers.

SHARING NEEDLES TO INJECT INTRAVENOUS DRUGS WITH AN HIV-INFECTED PERSON. The two necessary elements are present in this situation: infected blood and direct injection of that blood into the blood stream. During the process of injecting the drug blood is drawn into the syringe as the pump shaft is pulled in and out. Infected blood, then, can be mixed with the drug solution. If the syringe is passed to another individual and inserted in his or her body, infected blood from the previous person can be passed into the blood stream as part of the drug solution.

At first, this mode of transmission may appear contradictory in that HIV is taken *outside* the body first, then passed to another individual. This occurs, however, in the special context of a protective container — the closed confines of the syringe — where blood cells and virus are not exposed to the environment. In addition, it is generally done in a very short time, usually within minutes. Consequently, the blood cells remain alive and, with them, the HIV.

Prevention of this mode of transmission involves breaking the link between individuals via the syringe. IV drug users are encouraged first not to share needles. Some cities provide free sterile needles so that limited syringe availability is not an issue. Alternatively, IV drug users are encouraged to clean their needles between administrations using a bleach solution.

ACCIDENTAL NEEDLE STICKS AMONG HEALTH WORKERS. On occasion, health workers, in emergency situations or in the process of medical laboratory work with HIV-infected people, have accidentally stuck themselves with potentially contaminated needles. As of early 1988 there had been 660 reported cases; of these, three have become antibody positive. Thus, the probability of becoming infected following an accidental needle stick or cut is rather low. However, the risk does exist and health workers have been advised to wear gloves during clinical procedures. In addition, new needles have been designed that make accidental sticks more difficult.

INTIMATE SEXUAL CONTACT WITH AN HIV-INFECTED PERSON. For most people this mode of transmission is the most likely source of HIV infection risk. The risk differs, however, depending on the particular sexual practice. Consequently, this group of possible HIV transmission modes must be divided into four groups: safer, less risky, risky and dangerous. The differences among these groupings relate closely to the likelihood that the two critical elements—HIV-contaminated body fluid and direct contact with a target site—are present. Epidemiological findings provide the necessary supportive data on differences in actual incidence.

SAFER SEXUAL PRACTICES. This group includes touching, dry kissing, masturbation on healthy skin, and oral sex on a man using a condom. In each of these cases there is no direct contact with sites where susceptible cells are readily exposed. In two of the cases (masturbation and oral sex on a man), potentially-contaminated semen is present but, with proper precautions, the risk remains low. These precautions involve, in the case of masturbation, ejaculation of semen away from the body or onto healthy, unbroken skin and, in the case of oral sex on a man, use of a condom to contain the semen.

LESS RISKY SEXUAL PRACTICES. This group includes vaginal intercourse with a condom, anal intercourse with a condom, and wet kissing. Vaginal and anal sex clearly involve potentially contaminated body fluids (semen, vaginal and cervical secretions and blood), but, by using a condom, the possibility of direct contact with potential targets of infection (macrophages or mucosal linings) is reduced. The condom must be used properly, however. The condom should be made of latex (not natural products), placed on the man's erect penis prior to penetration, used with a water-based lubricant (not a grease- or oil-based lubricant, which destroys the latex) and remain in place on the man's penis until it is withdrawn from the vagina or anus.

Wet kissing (open-mouth kissing with tongue and saliva contact) presents a potential risk because of the theoretical presence (albeit very low) of HIV in saliva and of the presence of macrophages in the mucosal lining of the throat. Because the concentration of HIV that can be isolated in saliva is extremely low, the estimated risk is very low from wet kissing.

RISKY. This group includes masturbation on open skin, oral sex on a man without a condom and oral sex on a woman. Following our usual logic, these practices involve the exchange of potentially-contaminated body fluids and the potential of direct contact with target sites in the throat and blood stream. Because of data from epidemiological studies, however, the risks associated with these practices are less than might be predicted. In Chapter 6 data from the San Francisco Men's Health Study was presented on the risks associated with anal intercourse. These researchers also analyzed the risk from oral sex. As Table 7.1b shows, those subjects in the study who practiced only oral sex had a frequency of HIV infection that was essentially the same as that for those subjects who reported no sexual relations during the previous two years. Further corroborative results of this type could result in the reclassification of the risk of oral sex, at least between men, to a less risky category. On the other hand, there is one case report that a man who practiced oral sex exclusively contracted AIDS. This report, however, is based on one individual's self-reported behavior, whereas the data in Table 7.1b are from a study of over 1,000 men.

DANGEROUS. This groups of sexual practices includes vaginal intercourse without a condom, anal intercourse without a condom, and oral-anal contact. Vaginal and anal intercourse involve body fluids that can potentially contain high concentrations of HIV and direct contact with target sites. Beside the theoretical considerations, ample epidemiological evidence (see Chapter 6) documents that vaginal and anal intercourse are associated with HIV infection. Oral-anal contact also involves the potential for infection, particularly because of the likely intermixing during oral-anal sex of vaginal or seminal fluids near the anus. The epidemiological evidence for this latter practice is not extensive; future studies may provide data that support the inclusion of oral-anal contact in the "dangerous" category or may lead to its reclassification.

FIGURE 7-1. Recommended safe sexual practices (in use at the University of California).

Who should be aware of safer sex?

EVERYONE. Community understanding of how AIDS is transmitted will help to dispel the myths about what causes, *and does not cause*, AIDS.

Who should practice it?

Anyone and everyone who is sexually active.

What is safer sex?

SAFER:

Abstinence ● Dry kissing ● Masturbation on healthy skin ● Oral sex with a condom ● Touching ● Fantasy

LESS RISKY:

Vaginal intercourse with a condom ● Anal intercourse with a condom ● Wet kissing

RISKY:

Masturbation on open/broken skin ● Oral sex without a condom ●·Oral sex on a woman

DANGEROUS:

Vaginal intercourse without a condom ● Anal intercourse without a condom ● Oral/anal contact

SUBSTANCE ABUSE:

Use of the following substances may cloud your judgement and lead you to do things you normally would not. Amphetamines (speed) ● Amyl Nitrite (poppers) ● Alcohol ● Marijuana ● Cocaine

SYRINGES:

Sharing needles to inject intravenous drugs is very risky and transmits the AIDS virus.

Figure 7-1 presents a summary of current recommended safe sex guidelines. These particular guidelines are from the University of California, Irvine's AIDS Education Project and, like most similar guidelines, are based on recommendations from the U.S.

Surgeon General and the Centers for Disease Control. Anyone who is sexually active is encouraged to follow the "safer" sexual practices (abstinence, dry kissing, masturbation onto healthy skin, oral sex on a man with a condom, touching and fantasy) or the "less risky" practices (vaginal or anal intercourse with a latex condom, wet kissing). Condoms should be made of latex and should be used only with water-based lubricants, ideally those containing the spermicide monoxynol-9 that kills HIV virus in laboratory studies. The use of drugs and alcohol is also not recommended because of the way these substances can confuse judgments.

8

FUTURE DIRECTIONS IN COMBATTING AIDS

Society's Response to AIDS
  Education
  Research
  Treatment

Future Directions for Biomedical Efforts
• Prevention of Infection
  Public Health Education
  Vaccines

Treatment of Infected Individuals
  Anti-virals
  Restoration of the Immune System
  Treatment of Opportunistic Infections and Cancers

A Final Note of Optimism: Time is on Our Side

I N THIS BOOK we have learned about AIDS in terms of the basic biomedical aspects.   In terms of the biomedical picture we have considered the virus (HIV), the immune system, the physical manifestations of AIDS, how the virus is transmitted, and how transmission can be prevented.   However, the fact remains that HIV infection is continuing to spread in many areas of the world, and there is currently no "cure" for the disease. How can our society respond to this disease, and what are the areas where we are likely to see activity and progress?

SOCIETY'S RESPONSE TO AIDS

As discussed in Chapter 2, infectious diseases do not simply affect isolated individuals. They affect individuals who are living in societies, and the spread of an infectious agent is also affected by the interactions of individuals within a society.   Therefore, in combatting infectious diseases it is important to consider society as a whole in planning solutions. This is particularly important for diseases such as AIDS, for which there is currently no cure or preventative vaccine. There are three equally important approaches for society to combat any disease including AIDS: *Education, research* and *treatment*.

> *Education* will play several roles in fighting the AIDS epidemic. Education of the general population about AIDS and HIV will demystify the disease and reduce irrational fears. This may help the development of rational public policies concerning HIV-infected individuals and AIDS patients, and it may also reduce the discrimination and prejudice that these individuals suffer. Education about AIDS and HIV among health care workers will improve the quality and sensitivity of care that they provide to AIDS patients. Finally, education in high risk groups is critical to reducing the spread of HIV.

> *Research* will be important in providing biomedical solutions to the disease itself. Research in such areas as the virology of

HIV and the immune system will provide clues for possible therapies and cures. Epidemiological research may give us more information about how the virus spreads in populations, and what kinds of public health measures might be effective in controlling the disease. Finally, clinical research will test and validate new therapies for the disease itself.

In terms of biomedical research on AIDS, remarkable progress has been made in finding and studying the virus itself. Currently, the lack of a convenient animal model system is a major stumbling block. Faster progress could be made in understanding the disease process and testing therapies if HIV caused a similar disease in experimental animals. However, HIV only infects man and higher apes such as chimpanzees; furthermore, the virus does not cause disease in chimpanzees. Several retroviruses similar to HIV have been found recently in monkeys (SIV), and one strain induces immunodeficiency in rhesus monkeys, so this may be a useful model system. However, monkeys are very expensive to maintain in laboratories, they are in short supply, and the use of primates in research is strongly opposed by some animal welfare advocates. Thus, other more convenient animal model systems are desirable. One possibility is cats: there are two retroviruses of cats that cause immunodeficiencies.

Treatment of AIDS patients and HIV-infected individuals is another task that society must carry out either in the governmental or private sectors. AIDS is a devastating illness in a physical sense, and it also frequently leads to great economic and social hardships. The large number of individuals likely to develop the disease in the future will greatly strain our current health care resources in terms of personnel, facilities and finances. Our society will need to develop the proper methods to provide the best care possible for future AIDS patients.

FUTURE DIRECTIONS FOR BIOMEDICAL EFFORTS

The biomedical community will focus on two major problems regarding AIDS: 1) *Prevention of infection* by HIV, and 2) *Treatment of infected individuals who develop symptoms of the disease.* This will involve participation of individuals working in many disciplines, ranging from public health through basic laboratory science, to clinicians who treat patients. Let's look at some of the areas where current and future efforts are likely to focus:

PREVENTION OF INFECTION.

Public health education. Educational programs targeted to members of high risk groups will be extremely important. These programs will be the key to making these individuals aware of the dangers that they face, and also to promoting changes in behavior that will lessen the risks. As described in Chapter 2, the experience with the syphilis epidemic earlier this century shows the effectiveness of proper public health measures. As also discussed in Chapter 2, public health measures effectively limited the last plague outbreak at the turn of this century — even at a time when there was no cure for the disease. This is quite analogous to our present situation with AIDS.

In the context of AIDS public health education has been strongly endorsed by the Presidential AIDS Commission. As discussed in Chapter 7, safer sex recommendations have been developed to reduce the risk of spreading HIV infection through sexual relations. It will be very important to develop effective programs of education and behavior modification to persuade high risk individuals (particularly male homosexuals, IV drug abusers and their sexual partners) to adopt safer sex practices. Addressing HIV infection in IV drug abusers is an extremely critical issue, since these individuals may ultimately be the conduit for spread of infection into the general heterosexual population. The current programs have not been successful and they are under-funded.

Development and implementation of public health measures targeted to IV drug abusers will be challenging. For instance, as mentioned in Chapter 7 there are pilot programs to distribute clean IV needles to drug addicts in order to reduce the risk that they will share a contaminated needle with someone else. However, such programs have been opposed by some people who argue that distribution of needles condones and encourages drug addiction.

Development of public health programs to combat AIDS will also require particular attention to ethnic groups. As described in Chapter 6, Blacks and Hispanics represent a disproportionate number of AIDS patients. This is particularly true for HIV-infected individuals who are IV drug abusers — more than 75% of AIDS patients who acquired the disease through IV drug abuse are Black or Hispanic. Public health programs targeted to these groups will be very important.

Vaccines. Ideally, the most effective prevention of HIV infection would be a vaccine that blocks virus infection in an immunized individual. Indeed, effective vaccines have been developed against most human viruses that cause serious diseases. Several different possible vaccines against HIV have been developed very recently, principally through state-of-the-art "gene splicing" (or recombinant DNA) techniques. These candidate vaccines are being tested in monkeys, and initial human trials have begun on at least two of them. The first trials will simply determine if individuals injected with the test vaccines produce antibodies against HIV and if they experience no other harmful side-effects. Once this has been established, then other trials will test if the vaccines are effective in preventing HIV infection. It should be noted that testing of a vaccine in humans will create some ethical dilemmas — these issues are already under consideration.

Even though experimental HIV vaccines are already being tested, there are some theoretical reasons as to why it may be difficult to develop an effective one. As discussed in Chapter 4, HIV has a unique ability to evade the immune system in an infected individual. Briefly, this results from 1) the high mutation rate of the virus, particularly in the *env* gene; 2) the ability of the virus to establish a latent state in some cells; and 3) the ability of the virus to spread by cell-to-cell contact. The object of a vaccine is to raise a protective immune response to the infectious agent. Since HIV evades the immune system so efficiently, there is some question as to whether a vaccine can actually prevent HIV infection in an immunized individual, even if that individual produces neutralizing antibodies.

Despite these theoretical difficulties, there has been some encouraging progress recently. Using the monkey virus (SIV) as a model system, a vaccine consisting of killed SIV virus particles has been prepared. When this killed virus vaccine was used to immunize monkeys, it prevented them from developing viral infection or immunodeficiency when they were later injected with live SIV virus. This raises hope that a similar HIV vaccine might also be effective.

TREATMENT OF INFECTED INDIVIDUALS

Biomedical efforts on treatment of HIV-infected individuals will focus on three main areas: 1) *anti-virals* that interfere with continued HIV infection; 2) *restoration of the immune system*; and 3) *treatments of opportunistic infections and cancers*.

Anti-virals. As described in Chapters 4 and 6, AZT, which is an anti-viral compound against HIV, is an effective drug in AIDS patients. The fact that this drug works means that agents that interfere with continued HIV infection in an AIDS patient will improve the clinical status. Recent trials also tell us that treatment of infected asymptomatic individuals with AZT is effective in preventing or delaying the development of clinical disease. Thus, great efforts are being made to develop other anti-viral compounds that will also block HIV infection. Ultimately, it may be possible to use several anti-virals in combination and completely block the spread of HIV infection in an individual.

As was discussed in Chapter 4, AZT works by specifically blocking DNA synthesis carried out by HIV reverse transcriptase. Other related compounds are also being tested to see if they specifically affect HIV reverse transcriptase. Such compounds might have equivalent anti-viral effects. If they have fewer side effects than AZT, they may be even more effective in treating HIV-infected individuals. Two such compounds are currently undergoing clinical trials: dideoxy cytidine (ddC) and dideoxy inosine (ddI). Preliminary results indicate that they are effective in reducing HIV in infected individuals, but they also have some side effects.

Other potential anti-virals may be developed that attack other viral "Achilles heels" — processes that are vital to the virus but which are not necessary for the survival of the host cell. There are actually nine or ten different genes carried by HIV that specify proteins necessary for the virus life cycle. Any of these viral proteins are potentially targets for new anti-viral drugs. For example, drugs that interfere with the *tat* or *rev* regulatory proteins might prevent virus spread. Basic research on the growth cycle of HIV and related viruses will be important in pointing out new anti-virals.

Another potential class of anti-virals is that which interferes with the ability of the virus to enter cells. If the virus entry process is inhibited, then spread of infection within an individual might be inhibited. As discussed in Chapter 4, HIV virus particles initially attach to cells by way of the cellular receptor for CD4 protein, which is imbedded in the surface of normal T-lymphocytes and macrophages. Recently, recombinant DNA techniques have been used to make large amounts of a part of pure CD4 protein. Test tube experiments have shown that if enough CD4 protein fragment is incubated with T-lymphocytes or macrophages, it can compete with the CD4 receptors on the cells and prevent subsequent infection with HIV. It is possible that this approach might be effective in people as well. Another compound that sparked great interest a year or two ago is called dextran sulfate. Test tube experiments showed that dextran sulfate can also block HIV infection by interfering with viral entry, although the mechanism of action is not understood. Dextran sulfate is currently licensed for use as a blood anticoagulant in other countries such as Japan, which means that the drug has been successfully tested in those countries for lack of side effects. However, clinical trials did not show dramatic results in the ability of dextran sulfate to reduce HIV in infected individuals. Thus interest in it has waned.

Recently, another compound has attracted considerable interest: GLQ223 or compound Q. This drug is derived from a Chinese herbal medicine and it kills HIV-infected cells in culture. The compound is being tested in standard clinical trials as well as in some informal trials. Early results suggest that the drug may have some serious neurological side effects (including coma). At this time there is no agreement on whether compound Q is effective in combatting HIV infection in people.

Restoration of the immune system. Most of the clinical symptoms in AIDS result from failure of the immune system due to depletion of T_{helper} lymphocytes. If the immunological defects can be repaired, then the disease might be arrested or even reversed. As discussed in Chapter 3, all cells of the blood (including those of the immune system) arise by division and differentiation from stem cells that are located in the bone marrow. This process is controlled by a complex series of growth factors that circulate in the body, as described in Chapter 3. Blood cell growth factors are currently the subjects of a great deal of research — they are important in many other diseases in addition to AIDS. Ultimately, it may be possible to use these growth factors to stimulate and regenerate the immune system in AIDS patients. Of course, it will be important to use these growth factors in conjunction with anti-virals. Otherwise continued HIV infection would destroy the immune system again. Another potential complication is that growth factors may directly or indirectly activate HIV from latently infected cells.

In addition to naturally occurring growth factors for the immune system, several artificial substances that may be able to stimulate immune system regeneration are also being developed and tested.

Treatment of opportunistic infections and cancers. The major practical problems for AIDS patients generally are the opportunistic infections (OIs) and cancers that result from the lack of immunological protection. Thus development of better therapies for these OIs and cancers will play an important role in improved treatment of AIDS patients.

In terms of opportunistic infections, it will be necessary to develop effective drugs for each different OI. Many of these infections were rather rare before the AIDS epidemic, since the causative agents generally do not cause disease in healthy individuals. As a result, little effort had been put into developing drugs for them. For example, at the current time there is no effective treatment to control *cryptosporidiosis* as an opportunistic infection. The only recourse right now is to treat the symptoms (diarrhea). Now much more effort will be focused on developing drugs for these OIs.

In addition to developing new drugs, improved methods of delivery are also being developed. As an example, pentamidine is one of two treatments used for PCP pneumonia. Intravenous treatment with pentamidine is the standard procedure, but many patients experience side effects from the drug. Recently researchers have found that inhalation of a pentamidine mist brings the drug directly to the lungs and is very effective in treating PCP pneumonia. At the same time, the side effects of the drug are reduced, since it is delivered only to the area of infection (the lungs) and not to other regions of the body that may experience side effects. Aerosol pentamidine is now also being used preventively in HIV-infected individuals who have low T helper lymphocyte counts, but who have not yet developed PCP pneumonia.

The cancers that result from HIV infection range from Kaposi's sarcoma to tumors of the immune system called lymphomas. These cancers are actually quite distinct diseases, and different therapies will be necessary for each of them. In the case of Kaposi's sarcoma, one experimental treatment involves use of a naturally occurring protein called alpha-interferon. Cancer researchers may also provide new therapies for the cancers associated with AIDS.

A FINAL NOTE OF OPTIMISM: TIME IS ON OUR SIDE

Many of the facts and statistics about AIDS in this book are quite frightening and depressing, especially since a "cure" has not been developed yet. Indeed, those who are suffering from the disease or at risk to develop it often express frustration at the apparent lack of progress in AIDS research. But let's look at some time scales to get a sense of perspective. First, as discussed in Chapters 4 and 6, the current estimates are that most HIV-infected individuals will develop AIDS with an average time between initial infection and disease symptoms of eight to ten years. Thus, new therapies and treatments that are developed in the next five or ten years may be able to help many of those who are currently infected.

Second, let's look at the rate of scientific progress in the AIDS epidemic. For comparison, let's consider two other diseases that have had great impacts on society — the ancient disease plague (Black Death) and the more recent disease polio (see Chapter 2). Table 8-1 shows a comparison of the time scales for fighting these diseases. Plague probably first caused major epidemics as early as the fifth or sixth centuries A.D., with the well-documented Black Deaths occurring in the fourteenth and following centuries A.D. The infectious agent, *Yersinia pestis*, was finally isolated in 1908. Effective therapy against the disease had to wait for the development of antibiotics in the 1940s. Polio was first recognized as an epidemic disease in the 1880s, and the infectious agent, poliovirus, was isolated in the late 1940s. Even after the virus was identified, there was no effective therapy for individuals once they became infected. Ultimately, the disease was brought under control by the development of the Salk and Sabin polio vaccines beginning in 1955. As for AIDS, the disease was first recognized in 1981, and the causative agent, HIV, was isolated in 1983-1984. By the end of 1986 the first partially effective anti-viral, AZT, was developed, and put

TABLE 8-1:   A TIME COMPARISON OF THREE EPIDEMICS

DISEASE	1ST DOCUMENTED EPIDEMIC	ISOLATION OF AGENT	FIRST THERAPY
Plague	560 AD	1894 (yersinia pestis)	1940s (antibiotics)
Polio	1885 AD	1909 identified 1949 isolated (polio virus)	1953 (Salk vaccine)
AIDS	1981 AD	1984 (HIV)	1986 (AZT partially effective)

into wide use in 1987. Thus, the rate of progress in AIDS research has actually been very rapid in historical terms.

The rapid progress in AIDS research largely reflects great advances in molecular biology, virology, immunology and bio-technology that have taken place over the last twenty years. For instance, the life cycle of retroviruses was worked out largely in the 1970s — after the discovery of reverse transcriptase. In terms of immunology, the understanding of the different kinds of lymphocytes (B verses T; Tkiller verses Thelper) is also quite recent. The techniques to identify the CD4 protein of Thelper lymphocytes are less than fifteen years old. It is difficult to imagine how much more serious the AIDS epidemic would be if it had struck twenty years ago before these advances. One program that provided a major boost to these fields was the "War on Cancer," a program launched by the U.S. federal government to conquer cancer with the same approach used for putting a man on the moon. While the "War on Cancer" has not been won yet, the program resulted in a great deal of research on retroviruses, and it heavily contributed to the development of recombinant DNA cloning technologies. This has been essential to the rapid achievements in AIDS research. The fact that biomedical research has advanced so rapidly in the last few years also makes us optimistic that new and more effective solutions to HIV and AIDS will be developed in the not-too-distant future.

EPILOGUE

In the preceding chapters we have focused primarily on the biomedical aspects of AIDS: what HIV is, how retroviruses operate, how the immune system works, how HIV affects infected individuals, how HIV is transmitted, and so forth. Throughout our discussions, however, we have made frequent references to the social aspects of AIDS: what particular groups and subgroups of people are disproportionately affected by the disease, how fears and irrationality have affected actions taken against those with AIDS (or those thought to be susceptible to AIDS), and how certain erroneous beliefs about AIDS transmission persist despite scientific evidence to the contrary. The social aspects of AIDS are not only as important as the biomedical aspects, but they can directly influence the biomedical outcome. These two aspects will thus continually shape each other.

A complete understanding of AIDS, therefore, requires that we consider a social ecological view: focusing on the interactions within and between individuals, groups, communities and even nations. The importance of integrating social and biomedical aspects of AIDS is evident when almost any issue is considered. The following are some examples that highlight visible social issues of the AIDS epidemic:

We have a test for exposure to HIV (see Chapter 4) that is actually available at no cost in many places. However, whether or not a person decides to take the test is heavily influenced by social factors such as: the extent to which the individual perceives him or herself to be vulnerable to the disease (and this is distinct from his or her actual vulnerability); the attitude and response of the person's community towards AIDS; and the possible losses of job, insurance or housing in case of a positive antibody test. Yet the data that result from testing is needed for the development of a rational policy to manage the AIDS epidemic. This contrasts with most other medical tests, for instance one for diabetes. In this latter case, social factors have much less impact on a decision to take the test. The issue of testing, therefore, raises fundamental social and legal issues in which the rights of the individual and community may conflict.

The reactions towards individuals with AIDS by those who do not have the disease are often based on prejudices and unanalyzed personal beliefs, and less on facts or knowledge. This is even true for health care professionals, whom we would expect to have greater knowledge and to be more accepting of scientific facts. There are many instances of lack of action, inappropriate action, overreaction, and on occasion unprofessional action, towards AIDS patients. Individual perceptions, attitudes, beliefs and prejudices play important roles in determining how people respond to rational information on AIDS, as well as how they act towards AIDS patients or those suspected of having the disease. The perception of risk, rather than the measured risk, appears to be more important in determining how a society reacts.

Funding for AIDS research, education, prevention and treatment programs is heavily influenced by political considerations. Currently, funding for these programs is provided by federal, state and local governments, which must constantly make decisions about the allocation of scarce resources. A good case can be made that initial funding for AIDS programs was slow because those affected by AIDS (so far) have largely been members of stigmatized groups: gay men, drug users, immigrants, Blacks and Hispanics. The original outbreak of Legionnaire's Disease (see Chapter 6) provides an interesting contrast. In this case, the disease affected a relatively small number of middle-class white citizens, but there was a much more rapid commitment of government funds and officially-expressed concern. The funding for new diseases is heavily influenced by political considerations. A rapid procedure for major funding of the investigation of new and urgent diseases still awaits development.

Health insurance has been a major issue in the AIDS epidemic. Health insurance rules and regulations result from an interplay among economic, medical, social and political interests. Health insurance companies are motivated by profit and would prefer to test all applicants and exclude all antibody-positive individuals, or charge them very much higher rates. This would result in a situation where AIDS patients have no health insurance.

This attitude contrasts with the insurance industry's approach towards other groups, such as tobacco smokers. Although smokers also have more health problems they are generally not excluded by insurance companies. Instead, the insurance industry's policies towards smokers reflect the basic theoretical principle of insurance: to spread the burden over everybody in order to lessen the burden and suffering of any individual. A long term and catastrophic illness, such as AIDS, can financially stress this principle of a shared burden and illustrates a national problem of insuring against catastrophic disease.

Finally, many AIDS patients rely on state or county medical assistance if they do not have (or lose) private health insurance. In general, in order to qualify for such assistance these individuals must have completely exhausted their own financial resources, which is often viewed by AIDS patients as punitive and humiliating. These rules reflect a societal tendency to attribute causes to events, particularly negative ones. Such attributions lead to value judgments about the "worthiness" of support for groups of individuals such as AIDS patients, and they divert attention from the actual medical needs. It is interesting to contrast these policies with the unqualified support and assistance given to victims of floods and earthquakes in which "fault" is not apparently an issue.

A subsequent edition of this book is currently in preparation, and it will also address in detail the social, psychological, legal, ethical and political aspects of AIDS. In the meanwhile, we encourage the reader not to minimize their importance, but to be mindful of how intertwined they are with the biomedical aspects of the disease. Our understanding of AIDS requires multiple perspectives; likewise, short-term and long-term solutions to the disease will require multiple efforts at all levels. Changing society's views about AIDS will assist biomedical investigations, just as new treatment or vaccine developments will affect the AIDS political environment.

In personal terms there are positive approaches that we can take to dealing with the AIDS epidemic. Because death is an inevitable part of all our lives, it is more productive to focus on wellness and quality of life than on illness and death. This applies both to those who have AIDS and those who do not — as well as people affected by cancer or other terminal illnesses. Like all major social changes, AIDS presents us not only with problems but also with opportunities on both biomedical and social levels. For example, we have already expanded our scientific knowledge of the immune system due to the efforts to understand AIDS. We have equal opportunites to make progress on social issues, for instance developing effective AIDS prevention programs. Such prevention programs could also be models for dealing with other health issues. AIDS is a crisis and an opportunity for social improvement: the challenge is to use the opportunities for greater personal, social and biological understanding.

GLOSSARY

AIDS. Acquired Immune Deficiency Syndrome is an incurable, infectious, viral disease resulting in damage to the immune system in otherwise healthy individuals.

AIDS antibody test. A test to determine if an individual has antibodies to HIV, the virus that causes AIDS. Presence of HIV-specific antibodies indicates that the person has been exposed to HIV and raised an immune response, but it does not tell if the person is still infected. The most common test is the ELISA test. A back-up test called the Western blot is also used.

Analytical epidemiology. Epidemiological studies that seek to identify and explain the causes of diseases.

Antibiotics. Compounds that are effective against infection by micro-organisms such as bacteria, fungi and protozoa. They are generally ineffective against virus infections.

Antibody. A protein produced by a B-lymphocyte that specifically binds a particular antigen. This leads to attack by the immune system.

Antigen. A molecule or substance against which a specific immune response is raised.

Anti-virals. Compounds that are effective in treating virus infections.

Asymptomatic AIDS carriers. Individuals infected with HIV who do not show any sign of disease. They may be capable of infecting others.

Azidothymidine (AZT). Also called Retrovir or zidovudine. An anti-viral that is effective in treating HIV infection and AIDS. It works by preferentially inhibiting the action of reverse transcriptase during HIV replication.

Bacteria. Small, single-cell microorganisms that can cause diseases.

B-lymphocytes. One kind of lymphocyte. B-lymphocytes secrete antibodies that are specific for particular antigens.

Case/control studies. A form of analytical epidemiology in which a group of individuals with a particular disease (the cases) are compared to a matched group of unaffected individuals (the controls).

Case reports. Reports and descriptions of an unusual disease occurrence in individual patients. Case reports are one form of descriptive epidemiology.

Causality. The factors contributing to the development of disease in epidemiological studies.

CD4 protein. A surface protein that is characteristic of T$_{helper}$ lymphocytes. It is also present on some macrophages. CD4 protein is the cell receptor for HIV.

Cellular immunity. Immunity involving T-lymphocytes (particularly T$_{killer}$ lymphocytes).

Circulatory System. The system of vessels that moves blood around the body, including arteries, veins and capillaries.

Cohort studies. A form of analytical epidemiology in which a group of individuals who share a particular risk factor for a disease are studied.

Cross-sectional/prevalence studies. Monitoring of a population for occurrence of diseases, and noting the time and kind of diseases. A form of descriptive epidemiology.

Dementia. Loss of mental function due to damaged brain cells and brain inflammation in AIDS-afflicted patients.

Descriptive epidemiology. Epidemiological studies that describe the occurrence of disease by person, place and time. Generally the first kinds of studies carried out in a new disease.

Endemic pattern. Patterns of continuous infection that allow epidemic diseases to remain present in populations.

Epidemiology. The study of patterns of disease occurrence in populations, and the factors affecting them.

Experimental/interventional studies. A form of analytical epidemiology in which a condition in a population is changed, and the effect on disease development is observed.

Fungi. Microorganisms that may exist as single cells or be organized into simple multicellular organisms.

Germ theory. The proven postulate (1546) that infectious bacterial, fungal or viral organisms cause disease.

Helper T-lymphocytes. T-lymphocytes that "help" T_{killer} and B-lymphocytes respond to antigens. Destruction of T_{helper} lymphocytes is the major problem in AIDS.

HIV (Human Immunodeficiency Virus) The virus that causes AIDS; previously called HTLV-III, LAV and ARV. The predominant form of HIV in North America, Europe and central Africa is called HIV-1. A closely related retrovirus found in Western Africa is called HIV-2.

Humoral immunity. Immunity involving B-lymphocytes and the antibodies they produce.

Immune system. The circulating cells and serum fluids in the blood that provide continuous protection from foreign infectious agents, activate wound repair, and eliminate toxins and waste products.

Immunological memory. The ability of the immune system to respond rapidly to a previously-encountered antigen with specific antibodies.

Incidence. The proportion of a population that develops new cases of a disease during a particular time period.

Incubation period. Asymptomatic HIV incubation in otherwise healthy individuals during which time the disease may be unwittingly transmitted.

Kaposi's sarcoma. A normally rare cancer that develops frequently in AIDS-afflicted patients.

Killer or cytotoxic T-lymphocytes. T-lymphocytes that kill target cells that they bind to.

Koch's postulates. A series of criteria used to establish that a particular microorganism causes a disease.

Latency. A state of virus infection in which the virus genetic material remains hidden in the cell, but no virus is produced. At a later time the latent virus may become reactivated. HIV can establish latent infection, particularly in macrophages.

Lentiviruses. A sub-class of retroviruses that HIV belongs to. There are lentiviruses that infect other species, including old world monkeys, sheep and cats.

Lymphadenopathy syndrome (LAS). Persistently enlarged lymph nodes or "swollen glands," sometimes an early sign of HIV infection that is progressing. Also called PGL (persistent generalized lymphadenopathy).

Lymphatic circulation. A second circulatory system that lymphocytes circulate through. Lymph channels drain fluid from tissues (lymph) into lymph nodes, where B- and T-lymphocytes are located. Antibodies or T-lymphocytes are produced in the lymphnodes in response to infection, and they enter the general circulation by way of other lymph channels.

Lymphocytes. Cells of the immune system that respond specifically to foreign substances. There are several kinds of lymphocytes. The two classes of lymphocytes are B-lymphocytes and T-lymphocytes.

Lymphoma. Cancer of the immune system.

Lytic infection. Infection of a cell by a virus that results in death of the cell. HIV infection of T$_{helper}$ lymphocytes is a lytic process.

Macrophages. One kind of phagocyte. Macrophages generally attack cells infected with viruses.

Non-lytic infection. Infection of a cell by a virus that results in production of virus, but survival of the cell. Most retroviruses normally carry out non-lytic infections. HIV infection of macrophages is non-lytic.

Opportunistic infections. Infections by common microorganisms that usually do not cause problems in healthy individuals. OIs are the major health problems for AIDS patients.

Pandemic disease. An infectious disease present on many continents simultaneously.

Parasite-host relationship. The interaction between populations of predator (virus) vs. prey (human population).

Phagocytes. Cells of the immune system that "eat" foreign cells or infected cells. There are two kinds of phagocytes: macrophages and neutrophils (granulocytes).

Prevalence. The fraction of individuals in a population who have a disease or infection at a particular time.

Primary immune response. The immune response that follows exposure to an infection or an antigen for the first time. There is a lag period before antibodies are produced.

Protozoa. Large single-cell microorganisms that can cause diseases.

Red blood cells (erythrocytes). Blood cells that are responsible for carrying oxygen and carbon dioxide to and from the tissues.

Reverse transcriptase. An enzyme that is unique to all retroviruses. It reads the genetic information of the retrovirus, which is RNA, and makes a DNA copy.

Secondary immune response. An immune response that follows exposure to an infection or an antigen that the immune system has already encountered. The strength of the response is greater, it occurs more rapidly, and it lasts longer.

T-lymphocytes. One kind of lymphocyte. Unlike B-lymphocytes, T-lymphocytes do not release antibodies, but they specifically recognize and bind foreign antigens. There are two main types of T-lymphocytes: T_{killer} and T_{helper} lymphocytes.

Vaccine. A killed or harmless microorganism that can induce an immune response to a disease-causing agent. This will confer protection against the disease-causing agent in uninfected people. This is the major preventative measure against viral infections.

Viral envelopes. Structures that surround some virus particles, resembling membranes around cells. Viral envelopes contain virus-specificied proteins that are important in binding cell receptors. Viral envelope proteins are major targets for the immune system.

Viruses. Small infectious agents. They are parasites that must grow inside cells.

White blood cells (leukocytes). All blood cells except red blood cells. Leukocytes consist of a variety of blood cells including lymphocytes, neutrophils, eosinophils, macrophages and megakaryocytes.

Xenophobia. Discriminatory fear of foreigners.

INDEX